MILADY®
STANDARD

TEXTURE

ANGLE

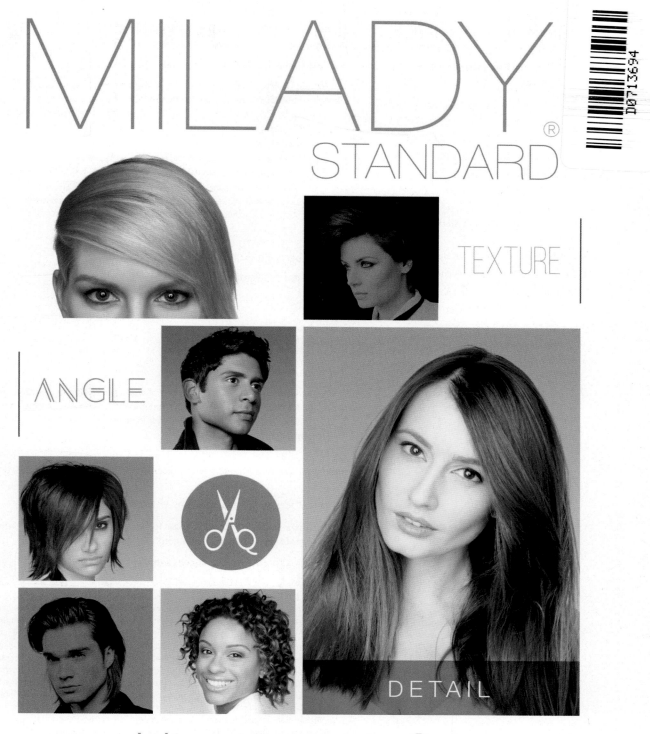

DETAIL

Haircutting System

CENGAGE
Learning®

Australia • Brazil • Mexico • Singapore • United Kingdom • United States

CENGAGE Learning

Milady Standard Haircutting System
Author: Milady

Editorial Contributors: Carlos Cintron, Skyler Marsh and Harry Garrott

Executive Director, Milady: Sandra Bruce

Product Director: Corina Santoro

Content Developer: Maria Lynch

Product Assistant: Harry Garrott and Michelle Whitehead

Senior Director of Sales and Marketing: Gerard McAvey

Marketing Manager: Elizabeth Bushey

Senior Production Director: Wendy Troeger

Production Director: Patty Stephan

Senior Content Project Manager: Nina Tucciarelli

Senior Art Director: Benj Gleeksman

Cover image(s): Photography by Yuki and Joseph Paradiso

For product information and technology assistance, contact us at
Cengage Learning Customer & Sales Support, 1-800-354-9706
For permission to use material from this text or product,
submit all requests online at **www.cengage.com/permissions.**
Further permissions questions can be e-mailed to
permissionrequest@cengage.com

Library of Congress Control Number: 2014950279

ISBN: 978-1-285-76970-7

Milady
20 Channel Center Street
Boston, MA 02210
USA

Cengage Learning is a leading provider of customized learning solutions with employees residing in nearly 40 different countries and sales in more than 125 countries around the world. Find your local representative at **www.cengage.com**.

Cengage Learning products are represented in Canada by Nelson Education, Ltd.

For your lifelong learning solutions, visit **www.milady.com**

Purchase any of our products at your local college store or at our preferred online store **www.cengagebrain.com**

Visit our corporate website at **cengage.com**.

Notice to the Reader

Publisher does not warrant or guarantee any of the products described herein or perform any independent analysis in connection with any of the product information contained herein. Publisher does not assume, and expressly disclaims, any obligation to obtain and include information other than that provided to it by the manufacturer. The reader is expressly warned to consider and adopt all safety precautions that might be indicated by the activities described herein and to avoid all potential hazards. By following the instructions contained herein, the reader willingly assumes all risks in connection with such instructions. The publisher makes no representations or warranties of any kind, including but not limited to, the warranties of fitness for particular purpose or merchantability, nor are any such representations implied with respect to the material set forth herein, and the publisher takes no responsibility with respect to such material. The publisher shall not be liable for any special, consequential, or exemplary damages resulting, in whole or part, from the readers' use of, or reliance upon, this material.

Printed in the United States of America
Print Number: 10   Print Year: 2022

Women's Haircutting with Finish

Men's Haircutting with Finish

Milady recognizes, with gratitude and respect, the many professionals who have offered their time to contribute to the *Milady Standard Haircutting System*, and wishes to extend enormous thanks to the following people:

Writing and Technical Expertise

Harry Garrott: for his dedication to the content and the many hours spent composing it into a single voice for the market to hear. For his tireless administrative support and positive attitude during the research and development of the product.

Carlos Cintron: VP of Education and Creative Director of KERATAGE for his editorial contributions to the content and passion for cosmetology education.

Skyler Marsh: Learning Leader and Cutting Specialist at Paul Mitchell The School Wichita and National Educator for John Paul Mitchell Systems, for his editorial contributions to the instructor and student facing materials and subject matter expertise at the photo–video shoot.

Photography

Joseph and Yuki Paradiso: For their brilliant photography and artistic vision, which resonates in every image.

On Camera Talent

Adam J. Federico: Creative Director of AJF Salon, Sacramento, CA

Christian Gaytan: Lead cutting specialist, Paul Mitchell The School Chicago, and John Paul Mitchell Systems National Educator, Chicago, IL

Stephen Adams: Moxie Hair Salon in Minneapolis, MN

Models: A big thanks to the fifteen models that graciously allowed us to cut, style, and transform them into their finished looks, in order to help educate future beauty professionals.

Off Camera Hairstylist

Courtney Nischan: Master Stylist, Hairroin Salon NYC, Oribe education team

Off Camera Hairstylist Assistant

Jessica Hayduk

On Camera Makeup

Doria Tremante

Alayne Curtiss

Product Providers

Burmax

ARROJO®: For generously providing backbar, and for on-camera talent use for the photo/video shoot.

Oribe®: For generously providing backbar, and for off-camera talent use for the photo/video shoot.

John Paul Mitchell Systems®: For generously providing on- and off-camera talent use for the photo/video shoot.

SAMVILLA®: For providing tools, implements, and supplies used on camera at the photo/video shoot.

Clothing

Kristina Collins Clothing: For graciously allowing us the use of timeless dresses and tops to bring our beautiful models' looks to life.

Tran Pham: For allowing us to borrow gorgeous vintage outfits to showcase our finished looks.

Clothes Styling

Alyssa Hardy: For her time and dedication as a fashion stylist at the photo shoot, outside of her normal duties at Milady, and for spending a great deal of time selecting and prepping outfits and jewelry accessories to create the overall presentation of our models' finished looks.

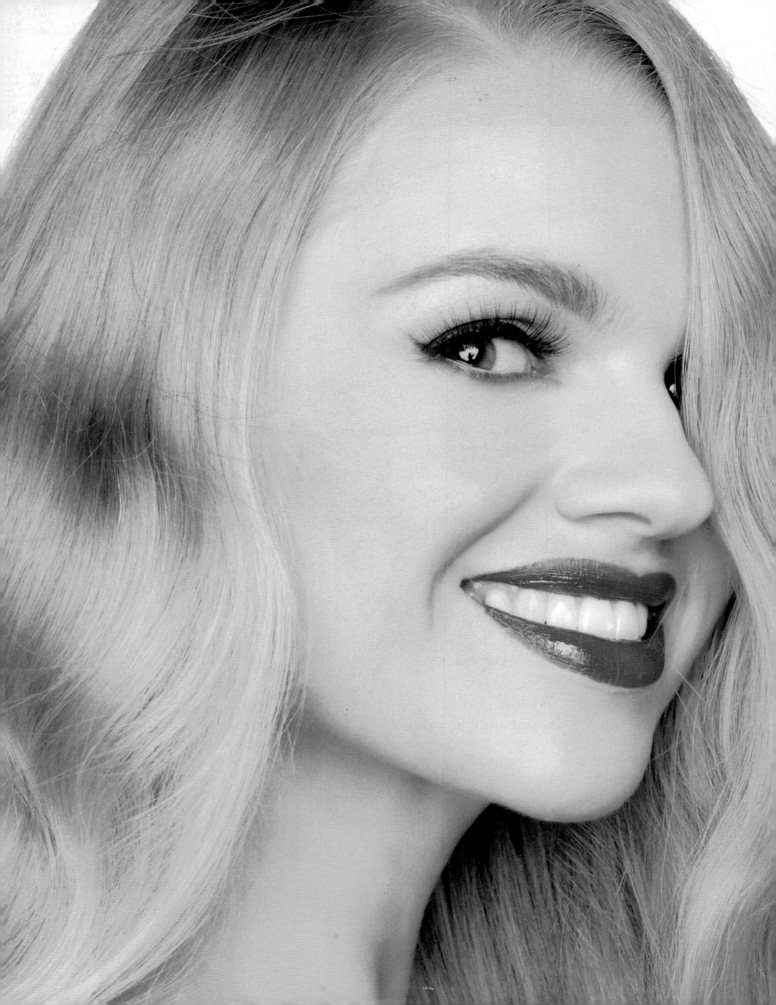

INTRODUCTION

Welcome to the *Milady Standard Haircutting System*, a standalone haircutting resource for the hairstylist in training as well as the experienced cosmetologist. The fifteen cuts that make up the system are designed to promote both conceptual and technical understanding of the founding principles of haircutting, through a systematic approach that reinforces core techniques in the process of adapting them afresh. By these means the new learner is introduced to the building blocks of haircutting, learning about both their consistency and their flexibility. They are asked to recognize not just when to use a technique or tool but how it might have been implemented differently. For the returning learner, this system affords the opportunity to revisit familiar haircuts and experience them in a new context, gaining a stronger understanding of the components involved and the creative potential that comes with that knowledge.

The cosmetology educator has a stake in this as well. In addition to the videos, instructor support slides, lesson plans, detailed step-by-step instruction, and practical grading sheets, the system as a whole comes with two pedagogical goals. The overarching one is to address and assess the technical aspects of haircutting in application. Haircutting is a skill, and this system is primarily here to build and strengthen that skill by means of repetition and revision, exposure and exploration. Connected with this drive toward expertise is the system's secondary mission: to help learners attain a level of conceptual understanding that allows them to clearly communicate their creative ideas, with classmates and guests alike. Developing this capacity has serious implications in the salon, from building guest confidence to upselling and merchandising, but it also has immediate benefits for the classroom. A common conceptual base built upon shared terminology can foster a rich learning environment – out of which understanding might grow into excellence.

Review of Foundational Building Blocks

Tools

The tools you will need to achieve the haircuts that follow are absolutely essential, as is your understanding of their proper use and care. Be sure to always have these tools in your kit: haircutting shears; texturizing shears; clippers; trimmers; sectioning clips; wide-tooth comb; barbering comb; styling or cutting comb; blowdryer; classic styling brush; paddle brush; small, medium, and large round brush; flat irons; and thermal irons. Knowing your tools will give you the ability to understand the best approach to cutting and styling any guest's hair. For the haircutting learner, this knowledge will allow you to be more confident when approaching your work, in addition to making you more marketable thanks to your expanded abilities.

Definitions are taken from *Milady Standard Cosmetology*:

- **Haircutting shears.** These shears, also known as *scissors*, are mainly used to cut blunt or straight lines in hair. They may also be used to slide cut, to point cut, or to implement other texturizing techniques.

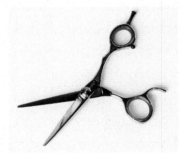

- **Texturizing shears.** Texturizing shears are mainly used to remove bulk from the hair. They are sometimes referred to as *thinning shears*, *tapering shears*, or *notching shears*. Many types of texturizing shears are used today, with varying numbers of teeth in the blades. A general rule of thumb is that the more teeth in the shears, the less hair is removed per cut. Notching shears are usually designed to remove more hair, with larger teeth set farther apart.

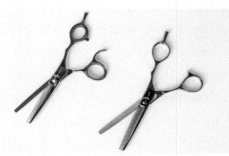

- **Clippers.** These are mainly used when creating short haircuts, short tapers, fades, and flat tops. Clippers may be used without a guard to shave hair right to the scalp, and with cutting guards of various lengths for the clipper-over-comb technique.

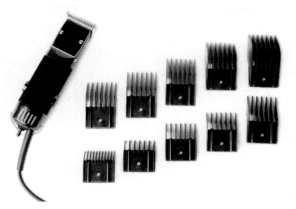

- **Trimmers.** These are a smaller version of clippers and are also known as *edgers*. They are mainly used to remove excess or unwanted hair at the neckline and around the ears and to create crisp outlines. Trimmers are generally used on men's haircuts and very short haircuts for women.

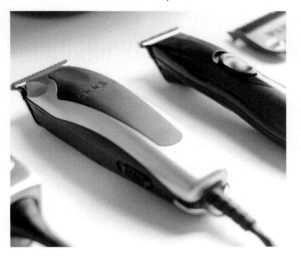

- **Sectioning clips.** These come in a variety of shapes, styles, and sizes and can be made of plastic or metal. In general, two types are used: jaw or butterfly clips and duckbill clips. Both come in large and small sizes.

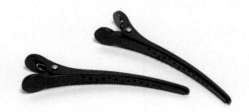

- **Wide-tooth comb.** This comb is mainly used to detangle hair. The wide-tooth comb is rarely used when performing a haircut.

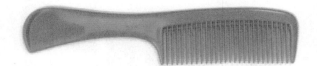

- **Barbering comb.** This comb is mainly used for close tapers on the nape and sides when using the scissor-over-comb technique. The narrow end of the comb allows the shears to get very close to the head.

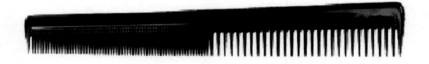

- **Styling or cutting comb.** Also referred to as an *all-purpose comb*, this tool is used for most haircutting procedures. It can be 6 to 8 inches (15.2 to 20.3 cm) long and has fine teeth at one end and wider teeth at the other.

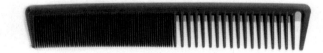

- **Blowdryer.** A blowdryer is an electrical appliance designed for drying and styling hair. Its main parts are a handle, slotted nozzle, small fan, heating element, and speed/heat controls. Some blowdryers also come with cooling buttons that are used to help set the hair. The temperature control switch helps to produce a steady stream of air at the desired temperature.

  - **Concentrator.** The blowdryer's nozzle attachment, this is a directional feature that creates a concentrated stream of air.

  - **Diffuser.** Another attachment that causes the air to flow more softly, and helps to accentuate or keep textural definition.

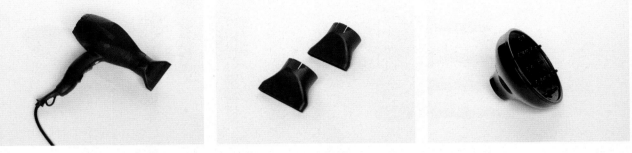

- **Classic styling brush.** A classic styling brush is a half-round, rubber-based brush. These brushes typically have either seven or nine rows of round-tipped nylon bristles. They are heat resistant, antistatic, and ideal for smoothing and untangling all types of hair. While they are perfect for blowdrying precision haircuts where little volume is desired, they are less suitable for smooth, classic looks.

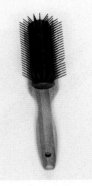

- **Paddle brush.** A paddle brush, with its large, flat base, is well suited for mid-length to longer-length hair. Some have ball-tipped nylon pins and staggered pin patterns that help keep the hair from snagging.

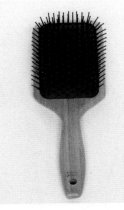

- **Round brushes.** Round brushes come in various diameters. The guest's hair should be long enough to wrap twice around the brush. Round brushes often have natural bristles, sometimes with nylon mixed in for better grip. Smaller brushes add more curl; larger brushes straighten the hair and bevel the ends of the hair. Medium round brushes can be used to lift the hair at the scalp. Some round brushes have metal cylinder bases so that the heat from the blowdryer is transferred to the metal base, creating a stronger curl that is similar to those produced with an electric roller. Always use the cooling button on the blowdryer before releasing the section to set the hair into the new shape.

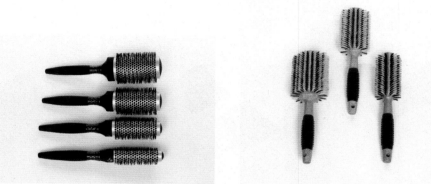

- **Flat irons.** Flat irons have two hot plates ranging in size from ½ inch to 3 inches (1.3 to 7.6 cm) across. Flat irons with straight edges are used to create smooth, straight styles – even on very curly hair. Flat irons with beveled edges can be manipulated to bend or cup the ends. The edge nearest the stylist is called the inner edge; the one farthest from the stylist is called the outer edge. Modern technology is constantly improving electric curling and flat irons by adding infinite heat settings for better control, constant heat even on high settings, ergonomic grips, and lightweight designs for ease of handling.

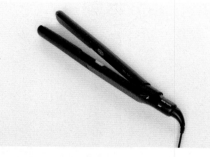

- **Thermal irons.** Thermal irons are implements made of quality steel that are used to curl dry hair. They provide an even heat that is completely controlled by the stylist. Electric curling irons have cylindrical barrels ranging from ½ inch to 3 inches (1.3 to 7.6 cm) in diameter.

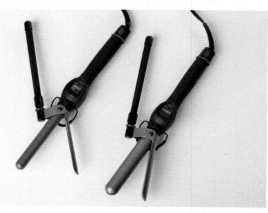

Products

Many haircuts, including those presented here, require the right products to produce the right finish, above and beyond the powers of you and your kit. Understanding the effects of products – from foams to hair sprays to thermal protection products – allows you to choose the right one depending on the texture of the hair both going into and leaving the service. This knowledge also allows you to recommend products to your guests for home maintenance, increasing your merchandising potential as it enhances your haircuts.

- **Foam.** Also known as *mousse*, foam is a light, airy, whipped styling product that resembles shaving foam. It builds moderate body and volume into the hair. Massage it into damp hair to highlight textural movement, or blowdry it straight for styles when body without texture is desired. Foam is good for fine hair because it does not weigh the hair down. It will hold for six to eight hours in dry conditions. Conditioning foams are excellent for drier, more porous hair.

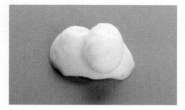

- **Gel.** A thickened styling preparation that comes in a tube or bottle. Gels create the strongest control for slicked or molded styles, and they add distinct texture definition when spread with the fingers. When hair is brushed out, gel creates long-lasting body. Firm hold gel formulations may overwhelm fine hair because of the high resin content. This is not a concern if fine hair is molded into the lines of the style and is not brushed through when dry.

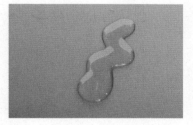

- **Liquid gels.** Also known as *texturizers*, liquid gels are similar to firm hold gels except that they are lighter and less viscous (more liquid) in form. They allow for easy styling, defining, and molding. With brushing, they add volume and body to the style. Good for all hair types, they offer firmer, longer hold for fine hair with the least amount of heaviness, and they give a lighter, more moderate hold for normal or coarse hair types.

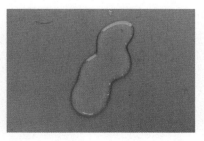

- **Straightening cream or gel.** When applied to damp hair (ranging from wavy to extremely curly) and blown dry, it creates a smooth, straight look that provides the most hold in dry outdoor conditions. Straightening gel counters frizz by coating the hair shaft and weighing it down. This is a temporary solution that will last only from shampoo to shampoo. Also, styles that use straightening gel may come undone in extremely humid conditions.

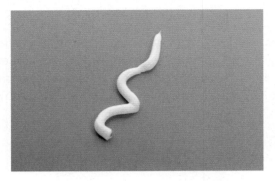

- **Volumizers.** When sprayed into the roots of fine, wet hair that is then blown dry, it adds volume, especially at the base. When a vent brush or round brush is used and the hair is not stretched too tightly around the brush, even more volume can be achieved. You may want to add a light gel or mousse to the rest of the hair for more hold, but be careful to avoid the roots and base of hair that has already been treated with volumizer.

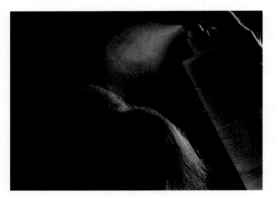

- **Pomade.** Pomade adds considerable weight to the hair by causing strands to join together, showing separation in the hair. Used on dry hair, pomade makes the hair very easy to mold, allowing greater manageability. It should be used sparingly on fine hair because of the weight. As a man's grooming product, pomade is excellent on short hair.

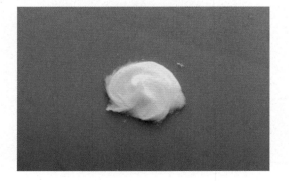

- **Silicone.** Also known as *serum*, silicone adds gloss and sheen to the hair while creating textural definition. Non-oily silicone products are excellent for all hair types, either to provide lubrication and protection to the hair during blowdrying, or to finish a style by adding extra shine. You can mix a couple of drops with most styling products before blowdrying. This application works best on dry, curly, and course hair.

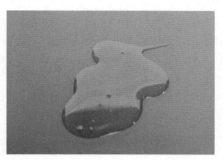

- **Hair spray.** Also known as *finishing spray*, it is applied in the form of a mist to hold a style in position. Hair spray is the most widely used hairstyling product. Available in both aerosol and pump containers, and in a variety of holding strengths, it is useful for all hair types. Finishing spray is used when the style is complete and will not be disturbed.

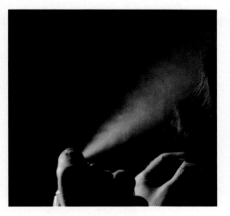

- **Thermal protection product.** Also known as *heat protection hair care product*, it is used on damp hair after you've applied styling product and before blow drying. Thermal protection products protect the hair from heat damage caused by thermal styling tools like blowdryers, flat irons, and curling irons. These products can come in a number of forms, including spray, cream, mousse, and serum.

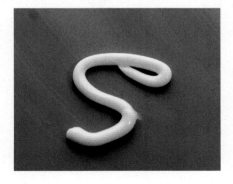

Principles of Haircutting

Lines, sections, partings, haircutting geometry, and reference points: these are the foundational concepts behind all haircuts. Once mastered over the course of this system, you will be able to confidently approach, perform, and diagram any haircut. As your skills develop and your repertoire of techniques expands, you will still find yourself continually returning to these core principles to help you analyze and tackle the project at hand.

- **Line.** A thin, continuous mark used as a guide. The two basic lines used in haircutting are straight and curved. The head itself is made up of curved and straight lines. When you cut lines in a haircut, the hair will fall into a shape.

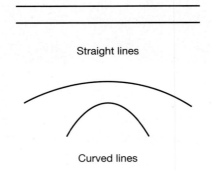

Straight lines

Curved lines

- **Section.** The working area that the hair is separated into prior to cutting.

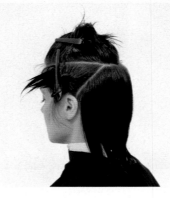

- **Parting.** The line dividing the hair at the scalp, separating one section of hair from another, creating sections.

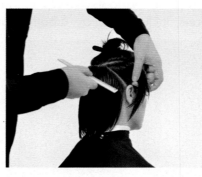

- **Geometry.** Geometry is used every day when cutting hair, however, some cuts – such as the A-Line and Perimeter Graduation – embrace the geometric and bring it to the fore. Elevation, distribution, and angles are the basis for creating geometry in haircutting, and understanding these principles will allow you to achieve different types of geometric haircuts, as well as many cuts not typically perceived to be quite so mathematical. As part of this process, you will also be able to distinguish between textured lines and geometric lines and understand how to apply them differently in various haircuts.

  - **Angle.** Created when the space between two lines or surfaces intersect at a given point. The angle at which you cut the line is what gives the hair direction and shape. Angles are important elements in creating a strong foundation and consistency in haircutting because this is how shapes are created.

  - **Elevation.** Also known as *projection* or *lifting*, elevation is the degree at which a subsection of hair is held, or elevated, from the head when cutting. Elevation creates graduation and layers, and is usually described in degrees. The most commonly used elevations are zero degrees, 45 degrees, and 90 degrees.

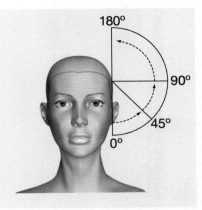

  - **Distribution.** Where and how hair is moved over the head.

- **Reference points.** Reference points on the head mark where the surface of the head changes, such as the ears, jawline, occipital bone, or apex. These points are used to establish design lines. An understanding of head shape and reference points will help you find balance within a design, so that both sides of the haircut turn out the same; develop the ability to create the same haircut consistently; and show where and when it is necessary to change technique to make up for irregularities (such as a flat crown) in the head form.

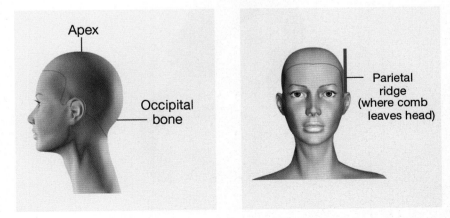

Foundational Haircuts

Once you understand the principles and geometry of haircutting, it is time to bring them to life in your first haircuts. The majority of haircuts are variations upon the four foundational cuts: the blunt, graduated, layered, and long-layered haircuts. As you gain experience in the techniques required to perform these haircuts, you will be able to apply your knowledge of haircutting principles to add complexity and experimentation to your work.

- **Blunt Haircut.** In a blunt haircut, also known as a *one-length haircut*, all the hair comes to a single hanging level, forming a weight line. The weight line is a visual line in the haircut, where the ends of the hair hang together. A blunt haircut is also referred to as a *zero-elevation cut* or *no-elevation cut*, because it has no elevation or overdirection.

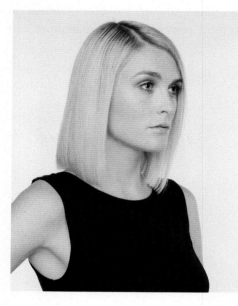

- **Graduated Haircut.** A graduated haircut is a graduated shape or wedge. This is caused by cutting the hair with tension, low to medium elevation, or overdirection. The most common elevation is 45 degrees. In a graduated haircut, there is a visual buildup of weight in a given area.

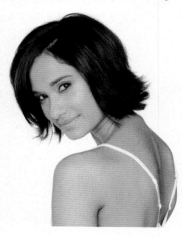

- **Layered Haircut.** A layered haircut is an effect achieved by cutting the hair with elevation or overdirection. The hair is cut at higher elevations, usually 90 degrees and above. Layered haircuts generally have less weight than graduated haircuts.

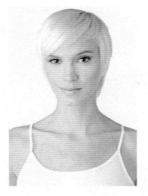

- **Long-Layered Haircut.** In a long-layered haircut, the hair is cut at a 180-degree angle. This technique gives more volume to hairstyles and can be combined with other basic haircuts.

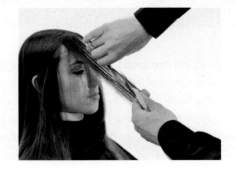

Haircutting Techniques

Advanced haircutting techniques are used to add definition to haircuts and to adapt any haircut to better suit your client's desires. These techniques work by creating texture, removing or shifting weight, instilling movement, ensuring balance, or maintaining a visual separation in haircuts.

- **Slide cutting.** A method of cutting or layering the hair in which the fingers and shears glide along the edge of the hair to remove length. It is useful for removing length, blending shorter lengths to longer lengths, and it is a perfect way to layer very long hair and keep weight at the perimeter. Rather than opening and closing the shears, you keep them partially open as you slide along the edge of the section. This technique should only be performed on wet hair, using very sharp shears.

- **Scissor-over-comb.** Also known as *shear-over-comb*, a barbering technique that has crossed over into cosmetology. In this technique, you hold the hair in place with the comb while using the tips of the shears to remove length. Scissor-over-comb is used to create very short tapers and allows you to cut from an extremely short length to longer lengths. In most cases, you start at the hairline and work your way up to the longer lengths.

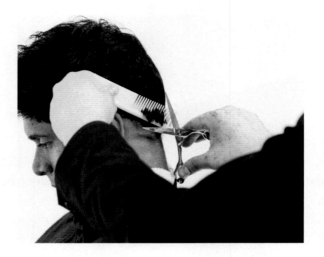

- **Texturizing.** The process of removing excess bulk without shortening the length. It can also be used to cut for effect within the hair length, causing wispy or spiky results.

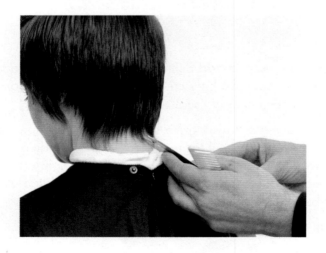

- **Point cutting.** A technique performed on the ends of the hair using the tips, or points, of the shears to create a broken edge. This can be done on wet hair to remove length and on dry hair to soften the line, remove weight, and create a seamless effect. It is very easy to do on dry hair because the hair stands up and away from your fingers. On wet hair (to remove length), hold the hair 1 to 2 inches (2.5 to 5.1 cm) from the ends. Turn your wrist so that the tips of the shears are pointing into the ends of the hair. Open and close the shears by moving your thumb as you work across the section. As you close the shears, move them away from your fingers to avoid cutting yourself. Move them back in toward your fingers as you open them. The more diagonal the angle of the shears, the more hair is taken away and the chunkier the effect. Basically, you are cutting points in the hair.

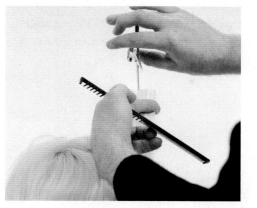

- **Notching.** Another version of point cutting, notching is more aggressive and creates a chunkier effect. Notching is done toward the ends. Hold the section about 3 inches (7.6 cm) from the ends. Place the tips of your shears about 2 inches (5.1 cm) from the ends. Close your shears as you quickly move them out toward the ends. If you are working on very thick hair, you can repeat the motion every $1/_8$ inch (0.3 cm). On medium to fine hair, place your notches farther apart. This technique can be done on wet or dry hair.

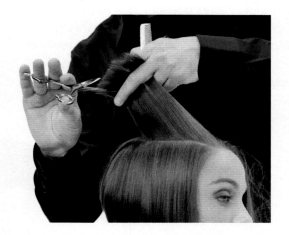

- **Effilating.** Also known as *slithering*, effilating is the process of thinning the hair to graduated lengths with shears. In this technique, the hair strand is cut by a sliding movement of the shears with the blades kept partially opened. Slithering reduces volume and creates movement.

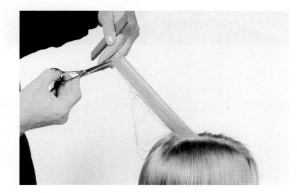

- **Slicing.** A technique that removes weight and adds movement through the lengths of the hair. When slicing, fan out the section of hair to be cut and never completely close the shears. Use only the portion of the blades near the pivot. This prevents removing large pieces of hair. This technique can be performed within a subsection or on the surface of the hair with haircutting or texturizing shears. To slice an elevated subsection, work with either wet or dry hair. When slicing to remove weight or on the surface of the haircut, it is best to work on dry hair because you can see exactly how much hair you are taking away.

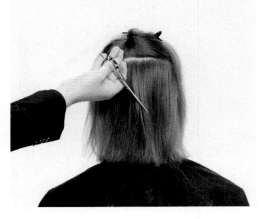

- **Carving.** A version of slicing that creates a visual separation in the hair. It works best on short hair (1½ to 3 inches [3.8 to 7.6 cm] in length). This technique is done by placing the still blade into the hair and resting it on the scalp. Move the shears through the hair, gently opening and partially closing them as you move, thus carving out areas. The more horizontal your shears, the more hair you remove; the more vertical, the less hair you remove.

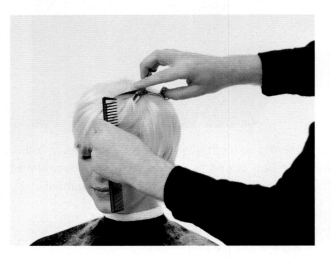

- **Cross-checking.** Parting the haircut in the opposite way that you cut it, at the same elevation, to check for precision of line and shape. For example, if you use vertical partings in a haircut, cross-check the lengths with horizontal partings. Always cross-check the haircut.

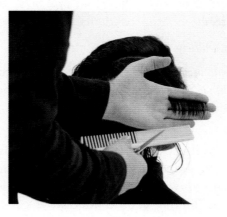

- **Disconnection.** When two lengths are not blended, instead being kept separate. This technique can be applied to both men's and women's haircuts.

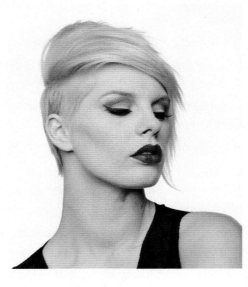

Bangs (Fringe) Cutting Techniques

The bang (fringe) area is the focal point of a haircut and can compliment many hairstyles. It is also a perfect choice for the client looking for change without sacrificing length. As you work through the *Haircutting System*, you will be instructed to choose a flattering fringe for your guest, if they would like a fringe. In those cases you should refer to the bang procedures here.

The following information is taken from *Milady Standard Cosmetology*:

The bang or fringe area includes the hair that lies between the two front corners, or approximately between the outer corners of the eyes. When cutting the bangs or fringe, be sure the hair is either damp or completely dry. Also, when combing and preparing to cut bangs or fringe, do not use tension; allow for the natural lift of the hair.

It is important to work with the natural distribution – where and how hair is moved over the head – when locating the bang area. Every head is different, and you need to make sure that you cut only the hair that falls in that area. Otherwise, you can end up with short pieces falling where they don't belong, ruining the lines of the haircut. When creating bangs (fringe), you do not always cut all of the hair in this area, and you only cut more if you are blending into the sides or the top.

There are five basic types of bangs (fringes):

- **Asymmetric Bang (Fringe).** Designed for all hair lengths; this bang style makes a statement and can vary from subtle to bold. Use shears.

  1. Start by placing an offset triangular section of hair at each corner of the eye.
  2. Take a ½-inch (1.3-cm) subsection at the narrowest part of the offset triangle, elevate at 90 degrees, and cut 2 to 3 inches (5.1 to 7.6 cm) (or longer) in length – this will become a stationary guide.
  3. Continue taking ½-inch (1.3-cm) subsections, elevate to 90 degrees, and overdirect to the stationary guide, or, for thick hair, overdirect to the previously cut section.
  4. Finish by blowdrying with a flat brush or comb. Using your comb for precision and angle, cut to desired length.

- **Side Swept Bang (Fringe).** Most commonly used on mid-length to long hair, this bang is worn on the side and works great for the client with a natural side part. Use shears or razor.

  1. Find the natural side part and take a subsection from the side part to the opposite corner of the hairline, forming an offset triangle.
  2. Starting at the side part (corner of the offset triangle), take a vertical section, elevate at 90 degrees, and blunt or point cut 3 to 4 inches (7.6 to 10.2 cm) in length – this will become a stationary guide. (The longer the guide, the longer the bang.)
  3. Take a ½-inch (1.3-cm), pie-shaped subsection and overdirect to the stationary guide. Continue taking ½-inch (1.3-cm), pie-shaped subsections and overdirecting to the stationary guide.
  4. Finish by cutting the perimeter at a 45-degree elevation from the face and cut on an angle, combing perpendicular to your section.
  5. Blowdry and remove weight by slicing or with texturizing shears. This will encourage the hair to sweep to the side.

- **Versatile Bang (Fringe).** Designed for all hair lengths, this type of bang can be worn on either side. Use shears or razor.

   1. Start by taking a (standard bang) triangle section at the top of the head.

   2. Take a ½-inch (1.3-cm) central vertical section, elevate at 90 degrees, and blunt or point cut 4 to 5 inches (10.2 to 12.7 cm) in length – this will become a stationary guide. (The longer the guide, the longer the bang.)

   3. Take a ½-inch (1.3-cm) subsection, elevate to 90 degrees, and overdirect to the center stationary guide. Continue taking ½-inch (1.3-cm) subsections and overdirecting to the center guide. Repeat on the opposite side.

   4. Finish by cutting the perimeter into a slight "V" shape.

   5. Blowdry and remove weight by slicing or with texturizing shears. Move from side to side and look for balance of weight.

- **Short Textured Bang (Fringe).** Most commonly used on short hair. Use shears or razor.

   1. Once you've completed your short haircut, start by taking a 1-inch (2.5-cm) horizontal section at the front hairline from recession to recession, elevate to 90 degrees, and point cut 2 to 3 inches (5.1 to 7.6 cm) in length.

   2. Blowdry the hair and detail the bang area visually. Using your cutting comb, elevate the hair and texturize with irregular deep point cutting. You may also use a razor to create a textured feel.

   3. Use your mirror and always make sure you achieve balance; the density of the hair will dictate how much texturizing is needed. Use the carving technique for separation and detail.

- **Square Bang (Fringe).** Designed for all hair lengths, this bang can be worn heavy or soft. Use shears.

   1. Start by taking a (standard bang) triangle section at the top of the head.

   2. Take a ½-inch (1.3-cm) subsection in the front hairline, comb to natural fall (with minimal tension), and elevate 2-fingers depth. Starting at the bridge of the nose, cut a square line and continue cutting until the corner of the eye. Repeat on the opposite side.

   3. Continue taking ½-inch (1.3-cm) subsections, elevate to 1-finger depth, and cut square following the guide from the previously cut section.

   4. For a heavy fringe, leave one length; for a softer fringe, layer using technique from the Versatile Bang (Fringe) (steps 2 and 3).

   5. Finish by blowdrying with a flat brush or comb. For heavy bangs, use your comb (for precision) and detail to desired length. For a softer fringe, remove weight by deep point cutting or with texturizing shears.

Haircutting Client Consultation Guidelines

A consultation is a conversation between you and your client when you find out what the client is looking for, offer suggestions and professional advice, and come to a joint decision about the most suitable haircut. A great haircut always begins with a great consultation.

The following information is taken from *Milady Standard Cosmetology*:

Begin the consultation by analyzing the client's freshly cleansed and unstyled hair for its natural behavior. Ask the client if there is anything he or she would like to discuss with you about his or her hair. Sometimes the client may ask you for your suggestions. Before recommending anything, you should consider the client's lifestyle and hair type. What is his or her lifestyle? How much time is he or she willing to spend on his or her hair every day?

Does the client want something that is classic or trendy? Problems may arise, for example, when a client with naturally curly hair is asking for a haircut that is really designed for straight hair. Will the client be willing to take the time to blowdry it straight every day? You will need to analyze hair density and texture, growth patterns, and hairline. If the client has hair that grows straight up at the nape and is requesting a short haircut that is soft and wispy at the nape, you should suggest other haircuts that will work with his or her hairline.

There are four characteristics that determine the behavior of the hair:

- **Hairlines and growth patterns.** Both the hairline and growth patterns are important to examine. The **hairline** is the hair that grows at the outermost perimeter along the face, around the ears, and on the neck. The **growth pattern** is the direction in which the hair grows from the scalp, also referred to as *natural fall* or *natural falling position*. Cowlicks, whorls, and other growth patterns affect where the hair ends up once it is dry. You may need to use less tension when cutting these areas to compensate for hair being pushed up when it dries, especially in the nape, or to avoid getting a hole around the ear in a one-length haircut. Another crucial area is the crown.

- **Hair density.** Hair density is the number of individual hair strands on 1 square inch (2.5 square cm) of scalp. It is usually described as thin, medium, or thick. The density of the hair will determine the size and number of the subsections needed to complete a cut. If there is too much hair in one subsection, it becomes difficult to see your guideline and to control the hair, because the hair is pushed away as you close the shears, producing an uneven line.

- **Hair texture.** Hair texture is based on the thickness or diameter of each hair strand, usually classified as coarse, medium, and fine. Density and texture are important because the different hair textures respond differently to the same type of cutting. Some hair textures need more layers, and some need more weight. For example, coarse hair tends to stick out more, especially if it is cut too short; fine hair, though, can be cut to very short lengths and still lies flat. However, if a client has fine (texture) and thin (density) hair, cutting too short can result in the scalp showing through (**table 1–1**).

	DENSITY		
TEXTURE	**THIN**	**MEDIUM**	**THICK**
Fine	Limp, needs weight.	Great for many cuts, especially blunt and low elevation. Razor cuts are good.	Usually needs more texturizing. Suitable for many haircuts.
Medium	Needs weight. Graduated shapes work well.	Great for most cuts. Hair can handle texturizing.	Many shapes are suitable. Texturizing usually necessary.
Coarse	Maintain some weight. Razor cuts not recommended.	Great for many shapes. Razor cuts appropriate if hair is in good condition.	Very short cuts do not work. Razors may frizz and expand hair. Maintain some length to weigh hair down.

- **Wave pattern.** The wave pattern, or the amount of movement in the hair strand, varies from client to client, as well as within the same head of hair. A client may have completely straight hair (no wave), wavy hair, curly hair, extremely curly hair, or anything in between.

Guest Preparation Procedure

After the consultation and before any professional cosmetology service can begin, the guest must be appropriately prepared for the haircutting service they are to receive. Guest draping is an important aspect of every overall service because it contributes to the guest's safety and comfort, in addition to the success of the haircut to come.

The following procedure is taken from *Milady Standard Cosmetology*:

1. Once the guest is comfortably seated in the shampoo chair, turn the guest's collar to the inside of their shirt, if needed.

2. Place a terry cloth towel, folded lengthwise and diagonally, across the guest's shoulders and cross the ends under the guest's chin.

3. Place a shampoo cape over the towel and fasten it in the back securely, making sure it does not touch the guest's skin.

4. Place another terry cloth towel over the cape and secure it in the front.

5. Proceed with the shampoo service as necessary.

6. Once the shampoo is completed, escort the guest back to your workstation.

7. Help the guest to get comfortably seated and, using towel two of the original draping, completely towel dry the hair. Once towel dry, pin long hair up and out of the way.

8. Remove the shampoo cape and towel one. Dispose of towels one and two properly.

9. Secure a neck strip around the guest's neck. Place and fasten a cutting or styling cape over the neck strip. Fold the neck strip down over the cape so that no part of the cape touches the guest's skin.

10. Proceed with the scheduled service.

System Haircuts

The following fifteen haircuts make up the *Haircutting System*, and appear grouped by length and then in order of increasing complexity, beginning with the basic Blunt Haircut. Additional information on the four foundational cuts — the blunt, graduated, uniform layered, and long-layered haircuts can be found in *Milady Standard Cosmetology*.

Women's Haircutting with Finish

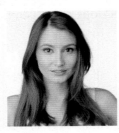

Blunt Haircut

The Blunt Haircut has many names: *solid form*, *one length*, *zero elevation*, and *bob*, to name a few. The Blunt Haircut is recognized as an all-time classic, marking a historic change from the total focus upon long hair that dominated prior to the twentieth century. For all the updates, trends, and variations, the original lines always look current and in style. The Blunt Haircut is adaptable to most textures, face shapes, and body types.

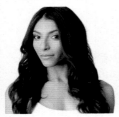

Long-Layered Haircut

While clearly similar to the Layered Haircut, this cut has some important differences designed for longer hair. In a long-layered haircut, increased layering is used, which features progressively longer layers. The guide here is an interior guide, beginning at the top of the head, and all remaining hair will be elevated directly up to match.

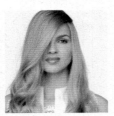

Perimeter Graduation

A combination of a one-length blunt haircut at the back with face-framing graduation. This haircut is ideal for the long-haired guest looking for change without layers. The perimeter is graduated then softened with deep parallel point cutting. Bangs (fringe) are optional.

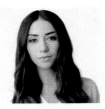

Long-Layered Overcut

A modern take on the Long-Layered Haircut, the Long-Layered Overcut gives the guest the option of having shorter layers at the top while still maintaining length. This technique can be finished with point cutting and slide cutting to give the haircut a combination of strength and softness while maintaining length.

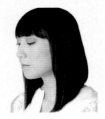

A-Line

This technique utilizes steep diagonal forward lines, creating a shorter length at the nape and a longer length at the sides. The angle at which the line is cut creates the A-line effect. This haircut can also be layered, depending on the texture of the hair. Bangs (fringe) are optional.

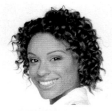

Layered Bob

A modern approach to a classic shape. This haircut is achieved by first establishing your length and then applying round layers with overdirection. It is finished by creating softness through texturizing while maintaining the bob line. Bangs (fringe) are optional.

Textured Graduation

This look is achieved by combining a vertical graduation technique with layers at the top. The haircut is finished with point cutting, creating texture, softness, and versatility.

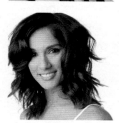

Mid-Length Layers

This haircut is ideal for shoulder- to collarbone-length hair. The longer uniformed layers in the interior are approached with deep point cutting or slice cutting, creating movements, and versatility.

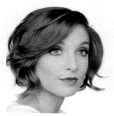

Graduated Haircut

Also known as the *bowl cut*, *wedge*, *stack*, and *emo cut*, the Graduated Haircut offers a tremendous amount of movement to the wearer. With its introduction in the 1970s, hairdressers were able to create inherent shape, volume, and movement, as well as the first of the "wash and wear" hairstyles. It is also an invaluable cutting technique for the guest with fine or thinning hair, giving them the desired look of fullness or thicker hair.

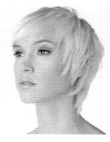

Uniform Layered Haircut

The Uniform Layered Haircut is the most popular and versatile of all cuts. The *rachel*, *farrah*, *mullet*, *pixie*, *shag*, and *afro* are just a few of the layered cuts that defined their eras, however it is a classic with no one particular defining look. The Uniform Layered Haircut lends volume, decreases weight, and adds internal texture and movement. These design factors are critical when considering the natural hair and desired style.

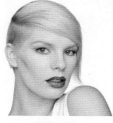

Graduated Undercut

This contemporary look is achieved by utilizing two separate cuts. The underneath is cut with short vertical graduation while the top is left longer and customized to suit the hair's texture, as well as the individual's lifestyle.

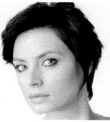

Disconnected Layers

A contemporary approach to a short haircut. Combining uniformed layers beneath a horseshoe section with a longer disconnected top. This look is then customized with an array of texturizing techniques for versatility and a modern edge.

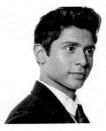

Short Texture

This classic masculine shape is modernized by combining scissor-over-comb and texturizing techniques. The end result is a versatile, low maintenance, cropped haircut suitable for men of all ages. Taper is optional.

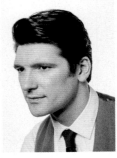

Square Layers

The distinct lines of square layers give this cut a defined edge that is undeniably masculine. This haircut can easily be transformed from business to casual, creating options for the contemporary male.

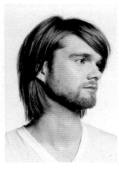

Versatile Movement

Designed for mid-length and shorter hair, the versatility of this haircut comes from the approach of the layering and the texturizing. The combination of strength and texture in the lines makes this style the perfect look for the fashion-forward male.

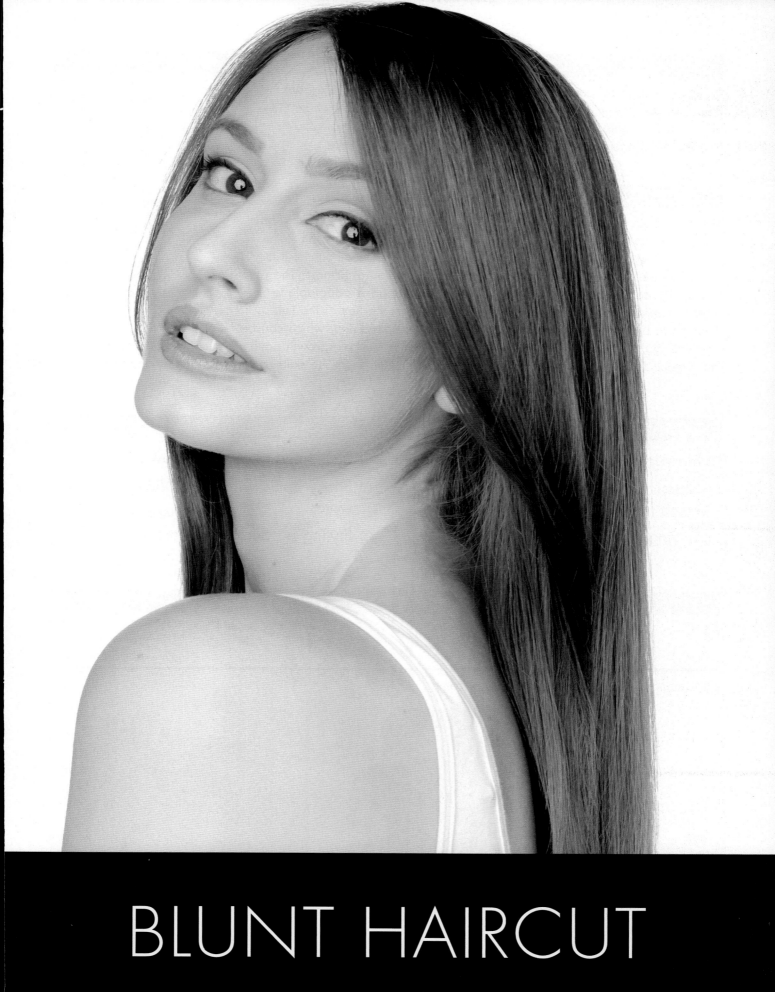

BLUNT HAIRCUT

After completing this section, you will be able to **perform** and **diagram** the Blunt Haircut. You will also **understand** and be able to **identify** whom the Blunt Haircut would be best suited for, what elevation it is cut at, and how that elevation affects the end result.

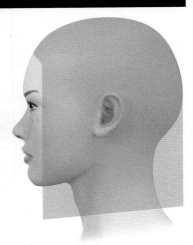

DESCRIPTION

The Blunt Haircut – also known as a *bob, one-length, one-level,* or *pageboy* haircut – is an all-time classic. In a blunt haircut, all the hair will fall to the same point, creating maximum density at the bottom of the silhouette. It is ideal for fine to medium texture hair, giving it the illusion of fullness. The cutting line can be horizontal, diagonal, or rounded and is adaptable to most textures, face shapes, and body types. Although the line of the cut appears to be simple, the success of the cut relies on precision, which can be anything but simple when working with a variety of hair types, growth patterns, and animated guests. All of the haircuts that follow in the Haircutting System will stem from the skills used in this first fundamental cut.

MATERIALS AND SUPPLIES

☐ Blowdryer

☐ Classic styling brush

☐ Cutting cape

☐ Cutting comb

☐ Haircutting shears

☐ Neck strip

☐ Sectioning clips

☐ Spray bottle with water

☐ Styling product

☐ Towels

☐ Wide-tooth comb

☐ Mannequin or model

STEPS TO HAIRCUT

❶ Carry out the **Guest Preparation Procedure**.

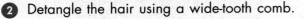

❷ Detangle the hair using a wide-tooth comb.

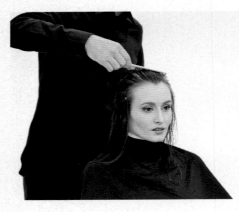

28

3 Part the hair in the center, from the front hairline through to the nape. Next, create two diagonal forward partings from the occipital to behind the ear, creating a ½-inch (1.3-cm) wide subsection. Make sure that your lines, sections, and partings are neat and balanced – use the mirror to ensure accuracy.

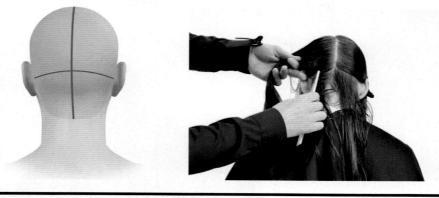

4 Angle the head forward slightly. Begin in the center on your nondominant side and, using the fine teeth, comb the hair to its natural fall. Cut your first line parallel to the diagonal forward parting, at zero-degree elevation.

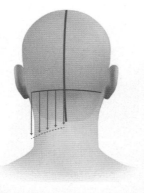
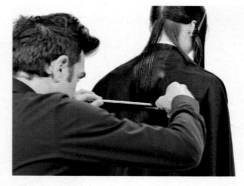

5 Repeat on the opposite side, starting the cut from the outer corner to the center, creating a slight arc-shaped line. Check for balance.

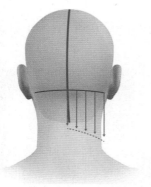
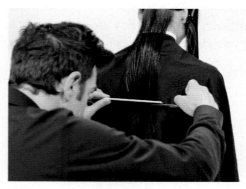

6 Now, from the top of the occipital to the top of each ear, create another set of diagonal forward partings. The head position will move up slightly, but the natural fall distribution and zero-degree elevation remain consistent. Cut parallel to your diagonal forward parting and follow the length of your guide.

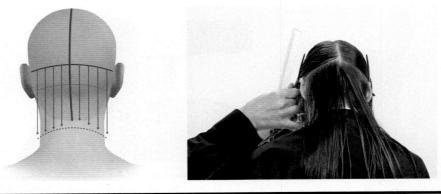

7 Position the guest's head upright. Beginning just below the crown and extending to the front hairline, create a horseshoe section. Starting in the rear of the horseshoe section, using the wide teeth, comb the hair over the previously cut hair to its natural fall (zero-degree elevation). Following your guide beneath, cut the line along the comb until you reach the side, just below the ear.

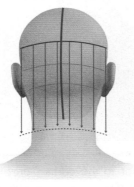
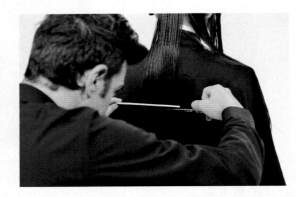

8 On the sides just behind the ear, continue to comb the hair to natural fall, cutting at zero degrees and parallel to the horseshoe parting. Pay close attention to the protrusion of the ear and tap the hair above the comb before you cut to release any tension.

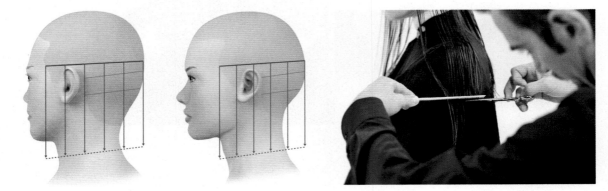

9 Repeat on the opposite side. Before moving on, stand behind the guest and check the lengths on both sides while looking in the mirror. Make any needed adjustments.

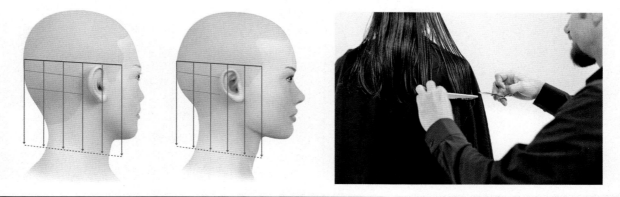

10 Take another set of subsections from the horseshoe above the crown to the front hairline. Starting at the back, comb the hair to natural fall and cut at zero degrees following your guide. When you reach the sides, continue the same technique as **step 8**.

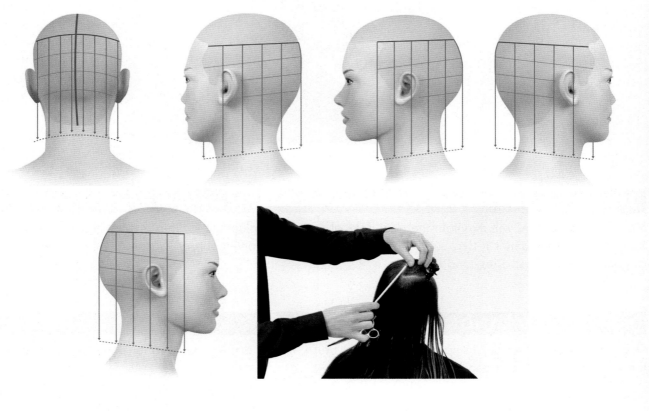

11 Release the remaining hair in the section and comb to natural fall. From the back, continue combing the hair to natural fall. Follow your guide and cut at zero-degree elevation.

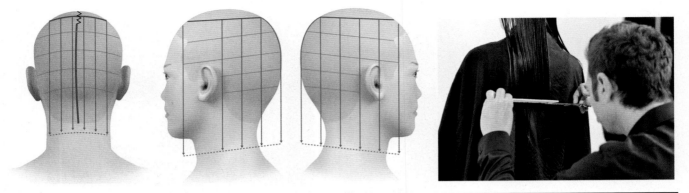

12 Perform a fringe consultation and cut the bangs as desired.

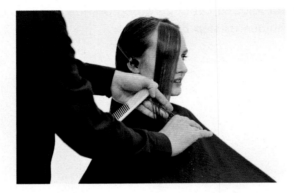

FINISH DESCRIPTION

When you style, you will maintain the neat lines of the classic blunt cut while directing and sectioning the hair in the same manner it was cut. It is a classic look with a contemporary twist that will work for a variety of guest face shapes, ages, and lifestyles.

FINISH PREPARATION

The hair will be blown dry using a classic styling brush. When dry, you will further define the perimeter of the haircut to reveal a strong blunt line.

13 Distribute styling product through the hair with your fingers and then comb through using a wide-tooth comb.

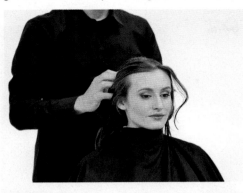

14 Start by removing any excess moisture from the hair and building volume at the root, by using a blowdryer and classic styling brush.

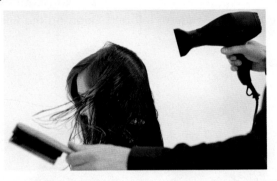

15 Once the excess moisture has been removed, section and part the hair in the same way it was cut.

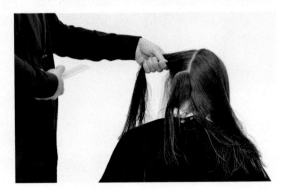

16 Blowdry each section straight and smooth and according to the amount of volume desired, using a classic styling brush. Do not use a round brush – it creates a bend in the ends of the hair, making it difficult to check the line.

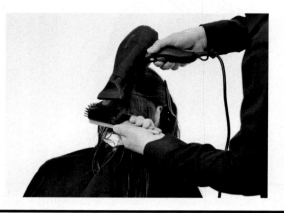

17 Once the hair is dry, check the line in the mirror: there should be an even horizontal line all the way around the head. Comb the hair to its natural fall and clean up the line as needed.

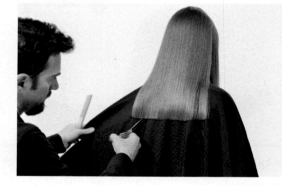

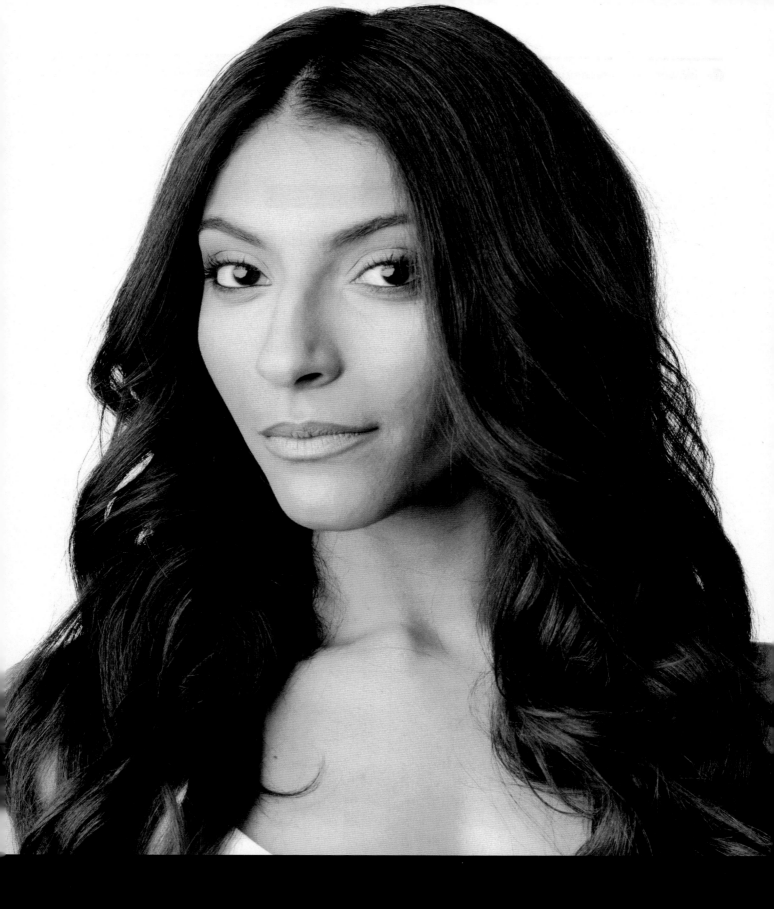

LONG-LAYERED HAIRCUT

LEARNING OBJECTIVES

After completing this section, you will be able to **perform** and **diagram** the Long-Layered Haircut. You will also **understand** the Long-Layered Haircut, why we need to learn what a layer does, and whom it would benefit the most.

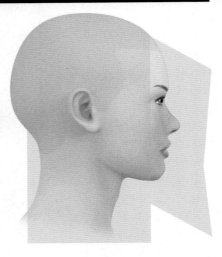

DESCRIPTION

The Long-Layered Haircut begins with cutting the perimeter line in the front, using some of the same techniques and principles seen in the Blunt Haircut. After the perimeter is complete, you will begin creating layers using a combination of overdirection, elevation, and a 45-degree finger angle along the front hairline and in front of the ear at the sides, as in Perimeter Graduation. Your guide for the interior layers and top will be a center profile section elevated to 90 degrees, extending from the occipital bone to the front hairline. The interior layers will be overdirected to match the length of your guide, which is then cut at 90 degrees.

MATERIALS AND SUPPLIES

- ☐ Blowdryer
- ☐ Cutting cape
- ☐ Cutting comb
- ☐ Diffuser
- ☐ Haircutting shears
- ☐ Neck strip
- ☐ Sectioning clips
- ☐ Spray bottle with water
- ☐ Styling product
- ☐ Towels
- ☐ Vent brush
- ☐ Wide-tooth comb
- ☐ Mannequin or model

STEPS TO HAIRCUT

1 Carry out the **Guest Preparation Procedure**.

2 Detangle the hair using a wide-tooth comb.

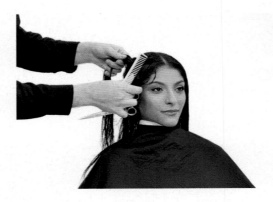

3 Begin by taking a central profile parting from the front hairline through to the nape. Then take two slightly diagonal forward subsections ½ inch (1.3 cm) wide from the occipital to behind the ear.

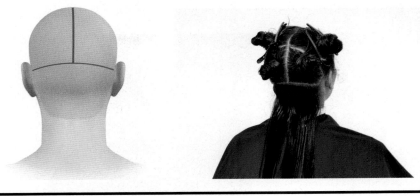

4 Tilt the head slightly forward. Starting in the center back, comb the hair to natural fall at zero degrees. Cut the line parallel to the parting to establish length. This will serve as your guide for the perimeter. The perimeter guide can be cut by either holding it with your fingers or a comb.

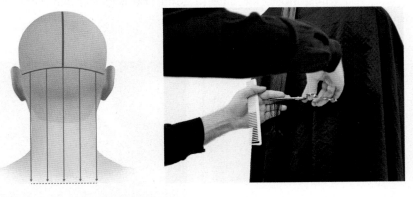

5 Take another ½ inch (1.3 cm) wide set of slightly diagonal forward subsections from the top of the occipital to the top of each ear. The head position will move up slightly, but the natural fall distribution and zero-degree elevation will remain. Cut parallel to the parting and following the length of your guide.

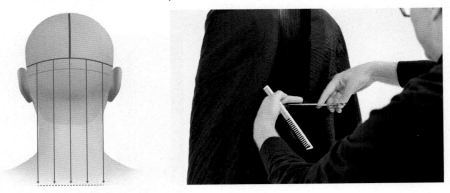

6 With the guest's head upright, take a horseshoe section from below the crown to the front hairline. Starting at the back of the head, comb the hair to natural fall and zero-degree elevation and cut the line following your guide. Check for balance as you move through the sections.

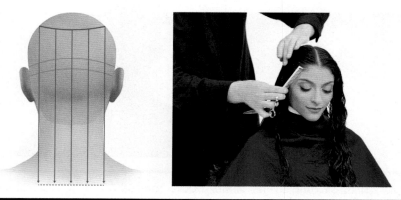

7 On the sides, comb the hair to natural fall and overdirect to behind the shoulder. Cut the line square to your guide. To do this, you will stand to the side to comb the hair to natural fall. Then step to the back and cut the line square.

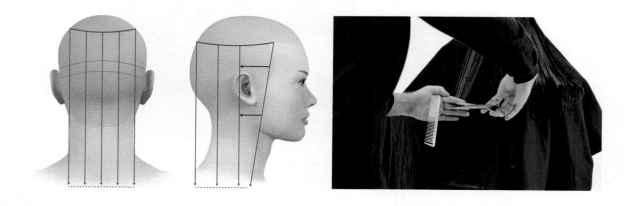

8 Repeat the same technique on the opposite side.

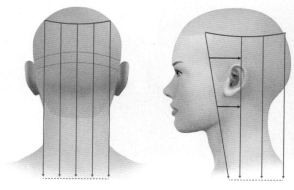
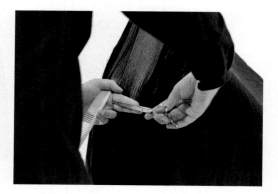

9 Continue this cutting technique with the hair inside the horseshoe until you have reached the profile part at the apex of the head or run out of hair to cut. Repeat on both sides.

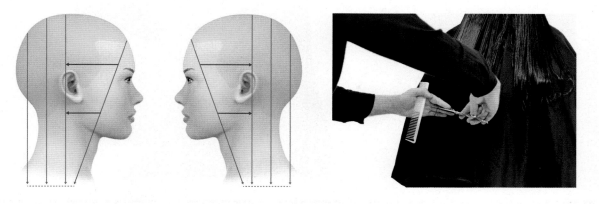

10 On the sides, take a diagonal back parting from the profile part to the top of each ear.

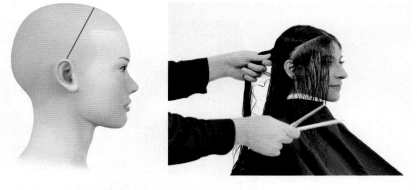

11 Standing to the front side of your guest, comb the hair parallel to your diagonal back parting, overdirect the hair forward, and, starting at the desired length, work your way from short to long through the perimeter.

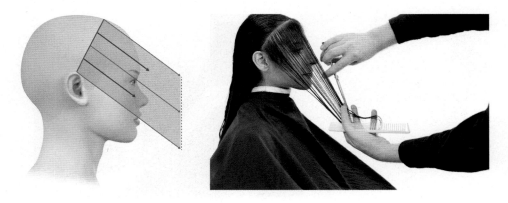

12 To keep the length on the sides from front to back, avoid cutting your corner at the sideburn area or just in front of the ear. Guests with long hair want to see their length at the front and back.

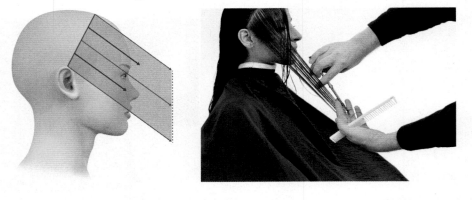

13 Take another diagonal back subsection. This time, extend to behind the ear, incorporating the hair from your first diagonal back subsection. Comb the hair parallel to the parting, overdirect the hair forward, and follow your guide.

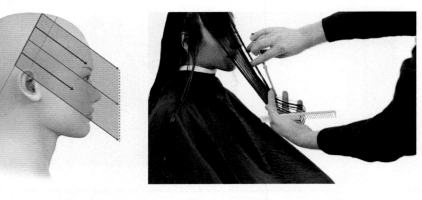

14 Although you are sectioning out and taking hair from behind the ear, this hair will not be cut. You will only be cutting hair from your corner, not what is behind the ear. Avoid overdirecting any hair beyond that point.

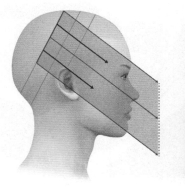
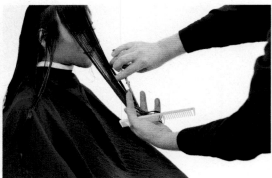

15 Continue taking diagonal back subsections, overdirecting toward the previous section, until you have reached the profile parting. At that point, you will be combing the hair at natural fall because you are cutting parallel to your line.

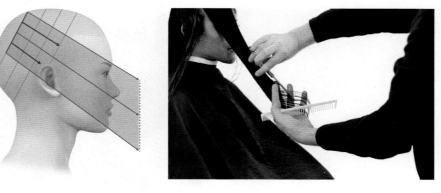

16 Repeat the same technique on the opposite side, paying close attention to body position, balance, and your corner.

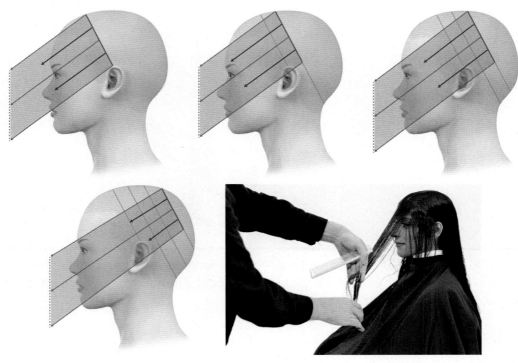

17 Once the sides are completed, check your balance by taking two diagonal forward partings at the top of the occipital to the back of each ear. The hair below your diagonal partings will be sectioned out of the way.

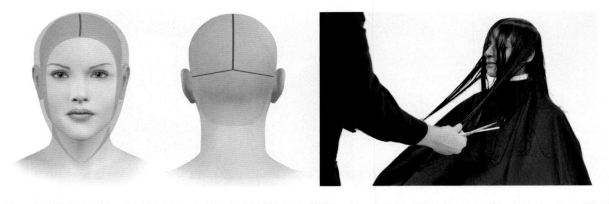

18 Starting at the front hairline, take a ½ inch (1.3 cm) profile section to the occipital bone, using your length from the chin as a guide.

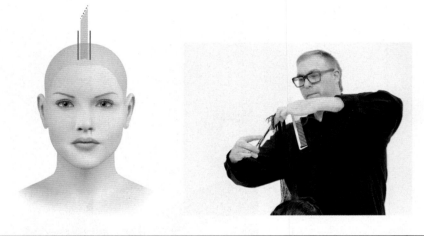

19 Elevate the profile section to 90 degrees and cut – as you work toward the occipital, increase your finger angle to blend the length from the back at the occipital. The layered profile section will serve as a stationary guide for your interior layers.

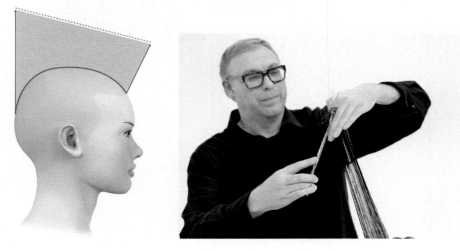

20 Below the crown and above the occipital, take a diagonal back subsection, elevate at 90 degrees, and overdirect to your center stationary guide. You should stand in front of the guide and overdirect the sections to your body, keeping your elbows up.

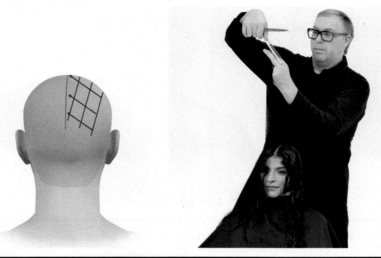

21 Continue taking diagonal back subsections, elevating up at 90 degrees, and overdirecting to the stationary center guide. Repeat until you have reached the front hairline section or run out of length. Make sure you are combing the hair diagonally back and up into the center.

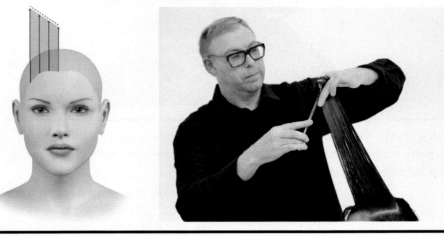

22 Repeat the same technique on the opposite side. Remember to switch body positions – stand on the opposite side and in front of your guide.

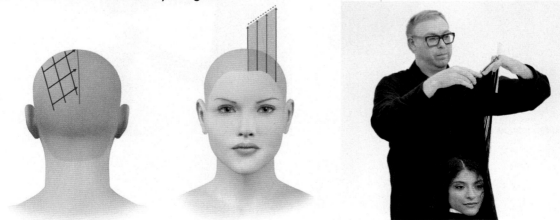

23 Cross-check the haircut by taking a horizontal section at the top and looking for an increase in length. Remember that when the hair travels to a stationary guide, it increases in length. The line should still be consistent, at a short to long angle.

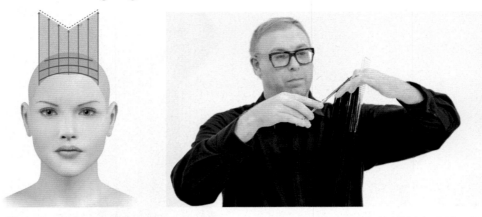

24 If more texture is desired, section the hair in the same manner in which it was cut and blowdry or diffuse.

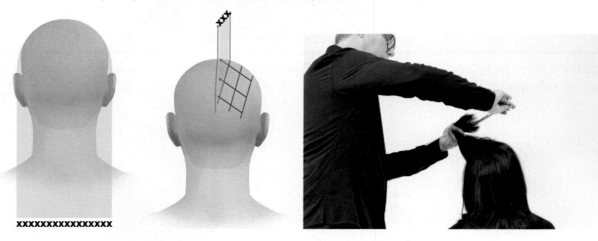

25 Once the hair is dry, detail the interior and perimeter using notching. Hold the section 3 inches (7.6 cm) from the ends and enter the hair parallel, using the entire length of the blade, so that you do not remove any length. Work in 1-inch (2.5-cm) panels.

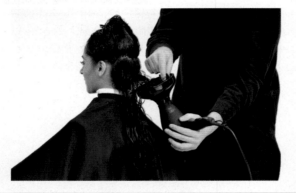

FINISH DESCRIPTION

The flowing layers of this shape come from the cutting technique used throughout the interior. It can be worn straight or in a full, voluminous look, and can be styled forward or back. It provides the guest with great versatility. In this layered shape, lengths progress from short layers through the interior to longer layers at the exterior. The layers provide textured volume. In this shape, the entire haircut is progressively layered – shorter lengths in the interior work toward longer lengths around the perimeter.

FINISH PREPARATION

When creating versatility within a haircut, products play a key role. When finishing any haircut, you must choose the finishing techniques and products that best support your guest's needs and wants for their style. Lengths move progressively from short layers in the interior to long layers on the exterior.

STEPS TO FINISH

26 Distribute styling product through slightly wet hair with your fingers and comb through with a wide-tooth comb. Always use products designed for your guest's hair texture.

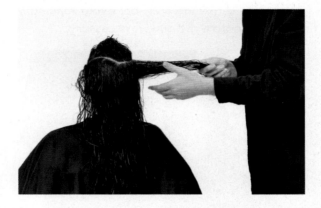

27 Position the hair the way the guest likes to wear it. Avoid placing a side part before diffusing; it will leave a line of demarcation. If the client wears it to the side, wait until the hair is 100 percent dry before placing a side part.

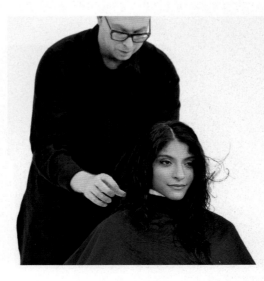

28 Attach the diffuser to the blowdryer, and have the guest tilt her head back or bend forward. Diffuse the hair by letting the hair sit on top of the diffuser and pulsing the dryer toward the scalp and then away, repeating until the section is dry.

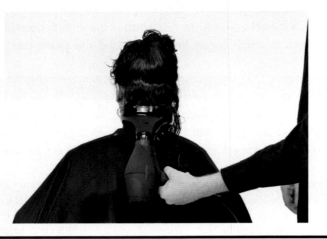

29 Avoid running your fingers through the hair until it is 100 percent dry; doing so will cause the hair to frizz. Once the hair is completely dry, shake the hair, but avoid running your fingers through or using a comb or brush. Use your fingers to separate the curl, if necessary.

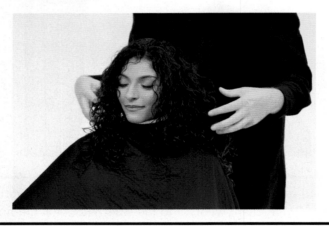

30 Finish by using a serum or shine product and evenly distribute it by gently scrunching the hair, trying not to disturb the curl.

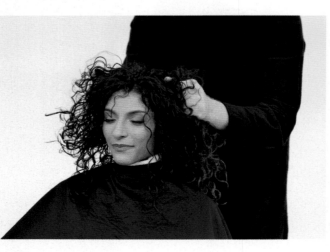

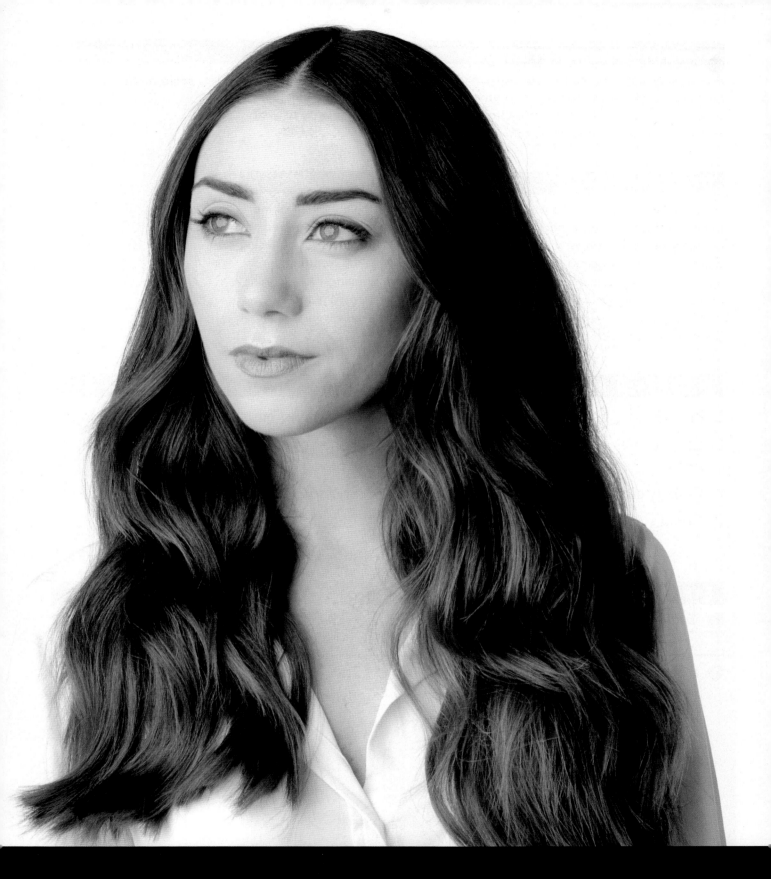

PERIMETER GRADUATION

LEARNING OBJECTIVES

After completing this section, you will be able to **perform** and **diagram** the Perimeter Graduation. You will also **understand** and be able to **identify** the differences between the Perimeter Graduation and the Blunt Haircut, as well as what makes it a graduation and why that matters.

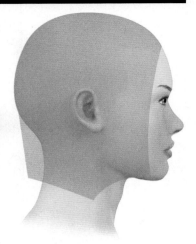

DESCRIPTION

A perimeter graduation is a combination of a one-length blunt haircut at the back with face-framing graduation. This haircut is ideal for the long-haired guest looking for change without layers. The Perimeter Graduation is cut using a stationary guide across the back – as you move toward the front hairline, the hair is overdirected back onto the stationary guide, creating more length in front. This length becomes the length we graduate to create the face-framing graduation. The perimeter is graduated, then softened with notching. Bangs are optional.

MATERIALS AND SUPPLIES

- ☐ Blowdryer
- ☐ Classic styling brush
- ☐ Cutting cape
- ☐ Cutting comb
- ☐ Flat iron
- ☐ Haircutting shears
- ☐ Neck strip
- ☐ Round brush
- ☐ Sectioning clips
- ☐ Spray bottle with water
- ☐ Styling product
- ☐ Towels
- ☐ Wide-tooth comb
- ☐ Mannequin or model

STEPS TO HAIRCUT

1 Carry out the **Guest Preparation Procedure**.

2 Detangle the hair using a wide-tooth comb.

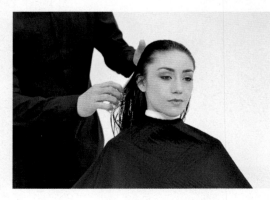

3 Place a profile parting from the center of the forehead to the nape. A center parting will allow the guest to style to either side. A side parting is optional. Make sure that your lines, sections, and partings are neat and balanced – use the mirror to ensure accuracy.

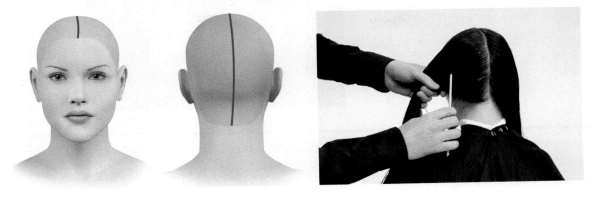

4 Place two slight diagonal forward partings from just above the occipital to the top of each ear, creating two large subsections. Comb the hair to natural fall and cut a blunt line parallel to the floor.

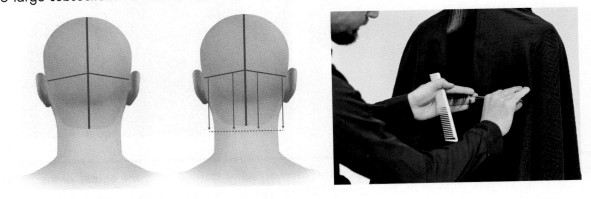

5 Place a horseshoe section from just below the crown to the parietal ridge on both sides. Starting at the back, comb the hair to natural fall (zero-degree elevation) and blunt cut parallel to the floor, following your guide from the previously cut section.

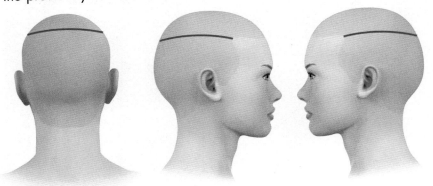

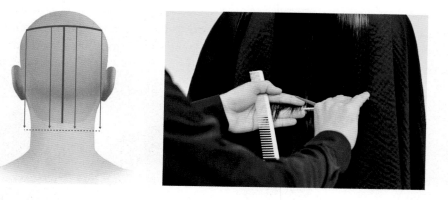

When transitioning to the sides, comb the hair down to natural fall, then overdirect the hair back to previous sections, cutting your line parallel to the floor and following your guide. Repeat the same technique on the opposite side.

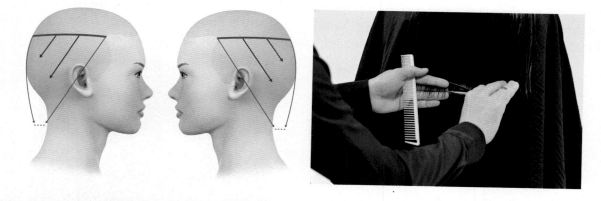

7 Release the remainder of the horseshoe section. Place a profile parting from the center of the forehead to the nape, then comb the hair to the natural fall. Be sure to separate the hair from the front and the back by placing a parting behind each ear. Using the guide from underneath, blunt cut your line parallel to the floor. Cross-check the length and clean up your line.

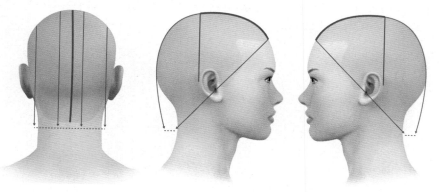

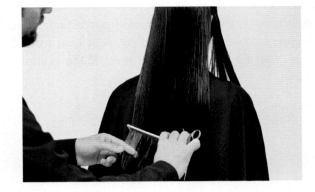

8. At the top, beginning at the center parting about 2 to 3 inches (5.1 to 7.6 cm) back from the front hairline, place a diagonal back parting to the top of the ear on both sides. Isolate all hair behind the parting out of the way. Starting at the left side, cut a visual guideline by using the sideburn area as your starting point. This will ensure that you maintain the corners of your length and avoid cutting your perimeter too short.

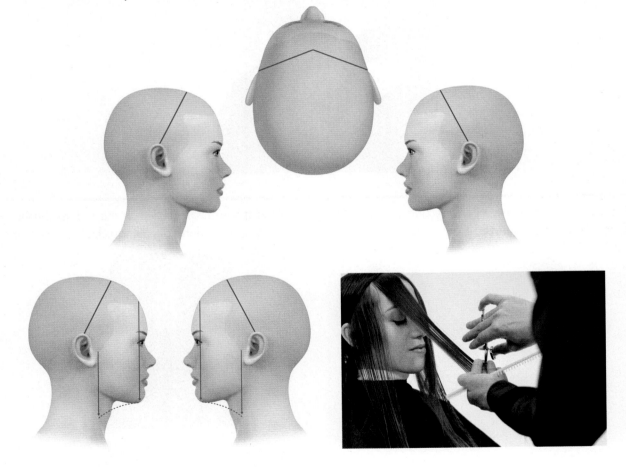

9 Comb the hair parallel to your diagonal back parting and overdirect forward. Elevate to 45 degrees from the face, angle your fingers toward the jaw, and cut your line, from the corner at the sideburn area to just below the jawline. Your body should be in front of the section you are cutting at all times. Repeat on the opposite side.

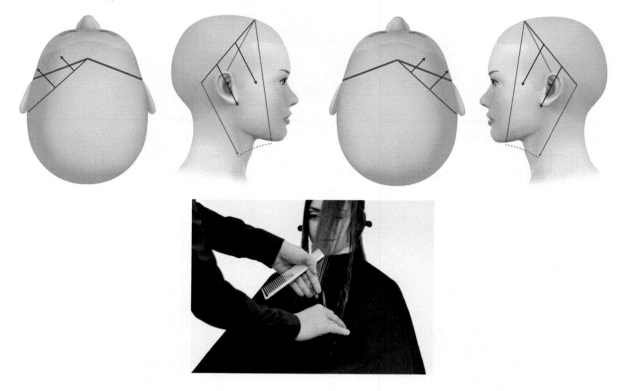

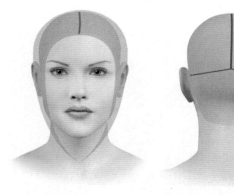

10 Check for balance between the guides for both sides before moving forward with the rest of the haircut. Once you have achieved your balance, resume on the top left side, behind your guide.

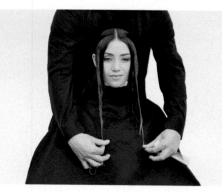

11 Take a 1 inch (2.5 cm) wide, pivoting diagonal back section from the center part to just behind the ear. Comb the hair parallel to your diagonal back parting, overdirect forward, and elevate to 45 degrees from the face and cut your line following your guide from underneath. Even though your partings are taken to just behind the ear, you will continue to only cut from the corner at the sideburn area up to the jawline.

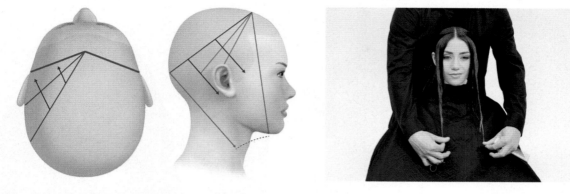

12 Continue this technique until you reach the center parting. At this point, you should be cutting the hair at natural fall because you are combing the hair parallel to the parting.

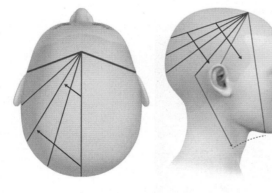
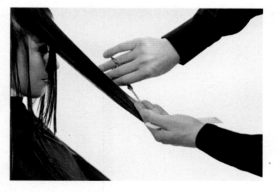

13 Switch body position and repeat the same technique on the opposite side.

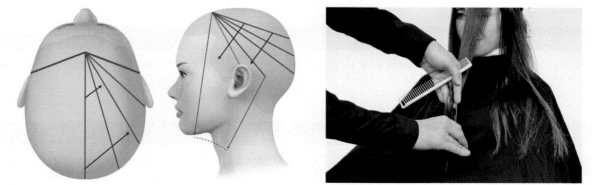

14 When dry, check your one-length line for accuracy and balance, utilizing the mirror. Detail your perimeter graduation by using notching, slicing, or carving if a softer look is desired. If the guest's hair is too long and overlaps the chair, have her stand up when detailing the length.

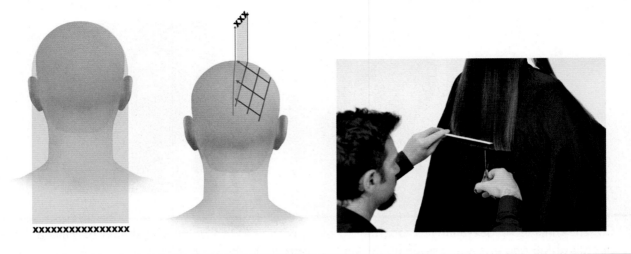

15 Perform a fringe consultation and cut the bangs if desired.

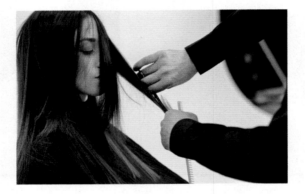

FINISH DESCRIPTION

This haircut is ideal for the guest who wants to maintain a one-length look. The face framing graduation gives the haircut movement and style.

FINISH PREPARATION

When blowdrying long hair, use lighter products like mousse or spray gels, giving the hair body and fullness. For a sleeker look, finish with a flat iron. Apply a serum or light oil for shine and separation.

16 Apply a thermal protectant followed by a mousse or light gel, combing through for even distribution.

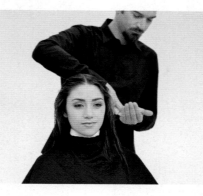

17 Section the hair exactly the way it was cut, then blowdry with a large round brush. For a sleeker look, a flat iron may be used once the hair is completely dry. Finish the haircut with a serum or light oil for shine and definition.

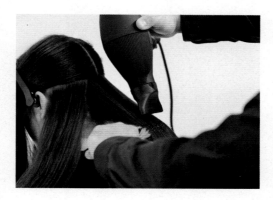

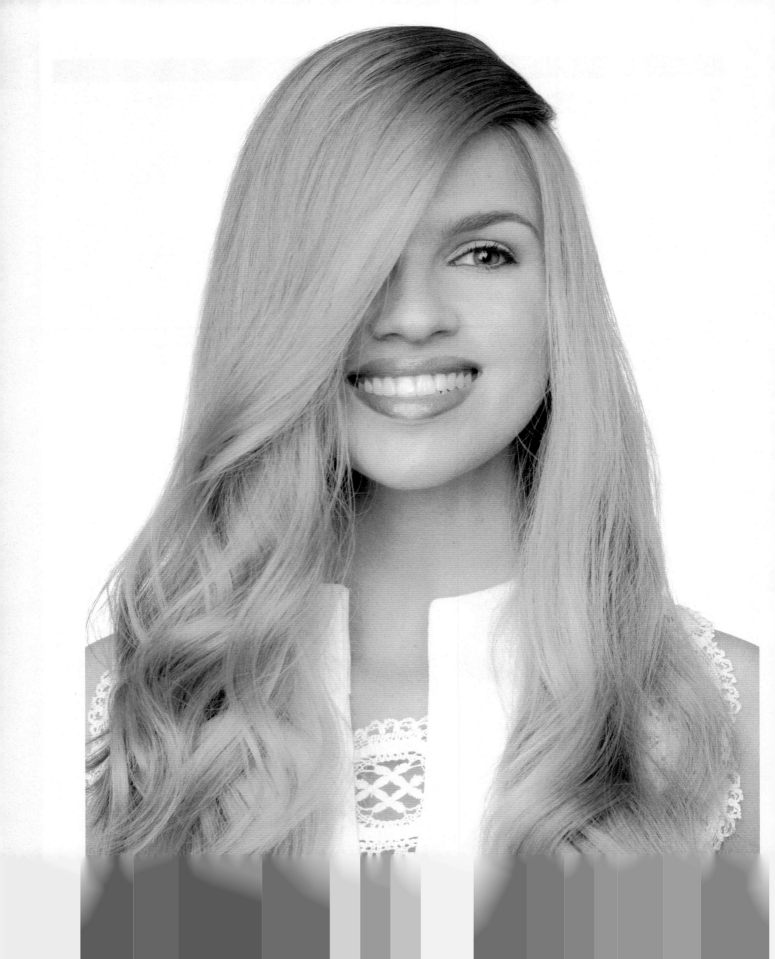

LEARNING OBJECTIVES

After completing this section, you will be able to **perform** and **diagram** the Long-Layered Overcut. You will also **understand** and be able to **identify** the differences between the Long-Layered Overcut and the Long-Layered Haircut, including using a stationary versus a traveling guide.

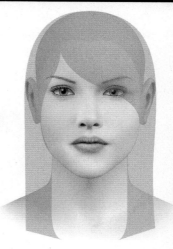

DESCRIPTION

A modern take on the Long-Layered Haircut, this look gives the guest the option of having shorter layers at the top and longer layers at the sides and back. The Long-Layered Overcut and Long-Layered Haircut both rely upon a combination of elevations and overdirections with a stationary guide to achieve layers. The stationary guide allows for the removal of weight while maintaining overall length. The Long-Layered Overcut differs by having shorter, more numerous layers in the top.

MATERIALS AND SUPPLIES

- ☐ Blowdryer
- ☐ Classic styling brush
- ☐ Cutting cape
- ☐ Cutting comb
- ☐ Flat iron
- ☐ Haircutting shears
- ☐ Neck strip
- ☐ Paddle brush
- ☐ Round brush
- ☐ Sectioning clips
- ☐ Spray bottle with water
- ☐ Styling product
- ☐ Towels
- ☐ Wide-tooth comb
- ☐ Mannequin or model

STEPS TO HAIRCUT

1. Carry out the **Guest Preparation Procedure**.

2. Detangle the hair using a wide-tooth comb.

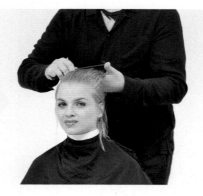

3 Place a horseshoe section from just below the crown to the parietal ridge on both sides of the head, then isolate the hair below the horseshoe with a sectioning clip. Make sure that your lines, sections, and partings are neat and balanced — use the mirror to ensure accuracy. At the top, create a band section by placing a part from the center of the forehead to the crown. On either side of the center part, section out a ¼ inch (0.6 cm) wide subsection of hair, creating a ½ inch (1.3 cm) wide band section.

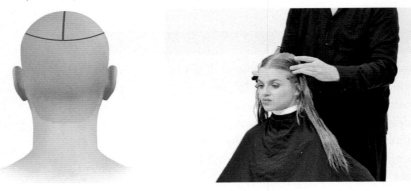

4 Elevate the hair up to 90 degrees from the head and cut a square line approximately 4 to 5 inches (10.2 to 12.7 cm) in length. This section will now become a stationary guide.

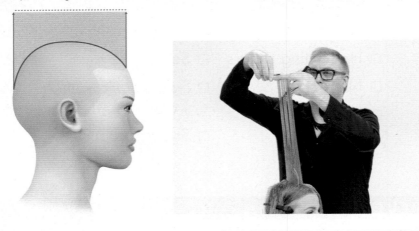

5 Standing parallel to your section, take a ½ inch (1.3 cm) wide vertical subsection. Elevate the hair up to 90 degrees from the head, overdirect to the center stationary guide, and cut square, following your guide from the previously cut section. Continue this technique until you have completed the first side.

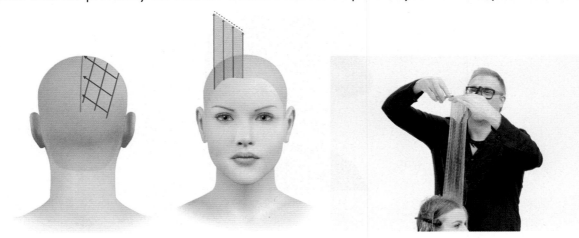

6 Repeat the technique on the opposite side.

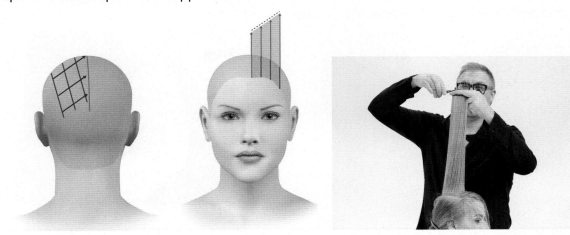

7 Cross-check your top sections horizontally. Because the hair was overdircted to the center, you will end up with a line that is slightly concave — do not square it off when cross-checking.

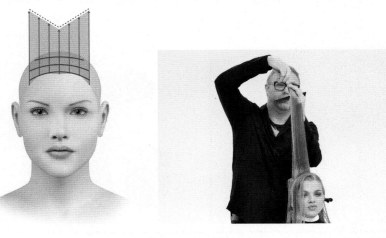

8 Release your isolated section and comb to natural fall. Create an arc section by taking a curved or diagonal forward parting from the top of each ear across the crown, and a horizontal parting from the top of each ear through the occipital. The hair in front of the ear and on top of the head will be isolated out of the way with clips.

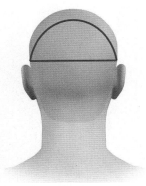

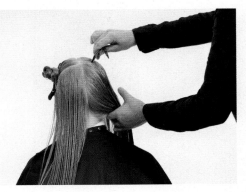

9 Place a center part from the front hairline to the nape. Take a ½ inch (1.3 cm) wide band section extending from the parting at the center lower crown to the nape.

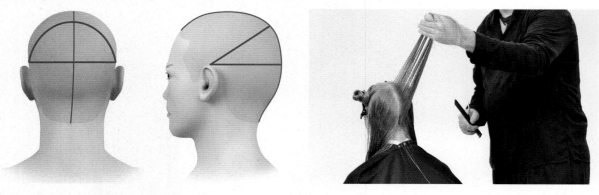

10 Elevate the hair to 90 degrees from the head and, using the length that was already cut in the crown as a guide, cut your layers, cutting from the top of the section down (from shortest to longest length). To ensure consistency in your cutting line and elevation, subdivide the length of your sections as you work if necessary.

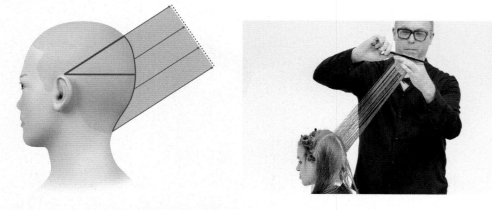

11 Take a ½ inch (1.3 cm) wide, pivoting section from the lower crown to the nape. Elevate the hair 90 degrees from the head and cut your layers from short to long, following your guide from the previously cut section. Be sure to subdivide the length of your sections as you work, if necessary. Continue the same approach until you have reached the parting at the top of the ear.

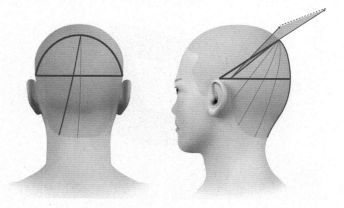

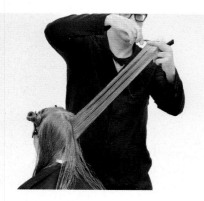

12 Repeat the technique on the opposite side.

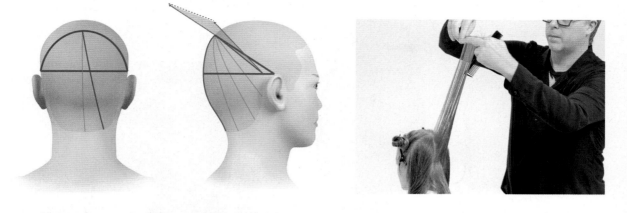

13 Beginning at the top of the crown, take a ½ inch (1.3 cm) wide, pivoting diagonal forward section to in front of the ear. Elevate the hair up to 90 degrees from the head, overdirect back, and point cut your line from short to long following your guide from the previously cut section behind the ear, working your way to the front hairline. Be sure to subdivide the length of your sections as you work if necessary.

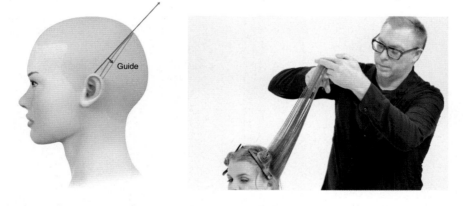

14 Continue taking ½ inch (1.3 cm) wide, pivoting diagonal forward subsections, elevating the hair to 90 degrees from the head, overdirecting back to the stationary guide behind the ear, then cutting your line from short to long following your guide from the previously cut section. Perform this technique until you have completed the side.

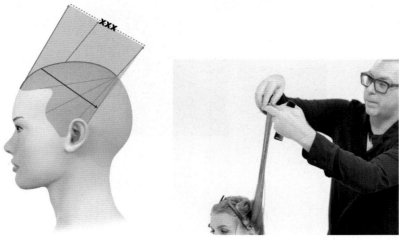

15 Switch body position and repeat the same technique on the opposite side.

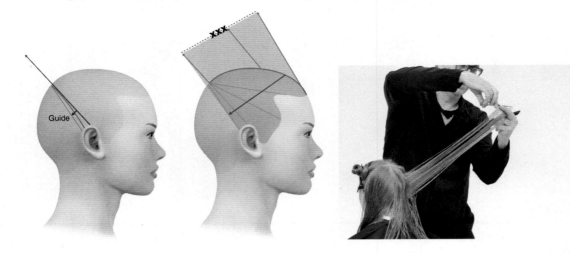

16 Once the layering is complete, stand at the back of the head, comb all of the hair to its natural fall, and cut your desired length square. Because the hair has been layered, it is not necessary to take sections to cut the length.

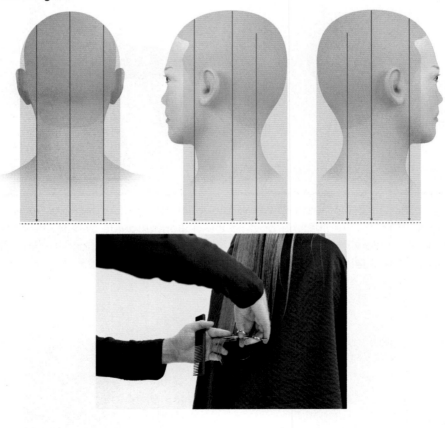

17 Begin detailing your length. Texturize the interior of the haircut by taking 1-inch (2.5-cm) panels and notching. This will soften your line and create a seamless effect for the layers.

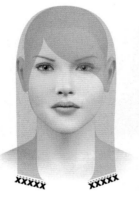

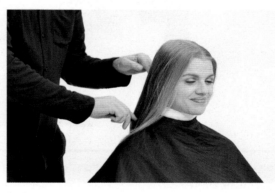

18 Because the top was cut with an inversion at the center, the guest has options to wear the hair with a center part or to either side. If needed, detail your perimeter with parallel point cutting and slicing.

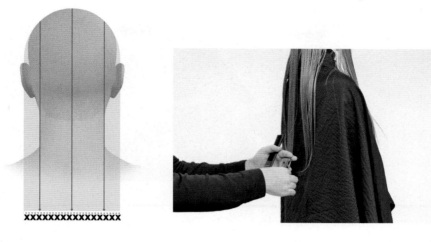

FINISH DESCRIPTION

This long haircut has some versatility: The top can be worn to either side or in the middle, and can be styled straight or with its natural texture. The cut is ideal for straight to wavy hair.

FINISH PREPARATION

Products play a key role in bringing out the versatility within a haircut, and understanding the hair's texture will make it easier to select the right styling aid. A volumizing mousse along with a thermal protectant will give fine to medium texture hair body and fullness; for thicker textures, gels or smoothing creams work best. Finishing products like waxes, serums, light oils, and aerosol hair sprays can be used to create definition, shine, and fullness.

19 Apply a volumizing mousse and a thermal protectant, comb from root to ends for even distribution.

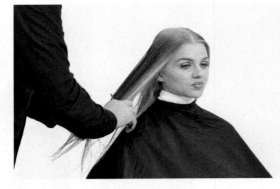

20 Blowdry the hair with a round or paddle brush. Once completely dry, take ½-inch (1.3-cm) panels and flatiron all of the hair if needed.

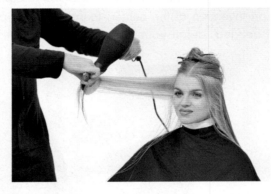

21 Apply a light wax or serum for shine, definition, and separation; finish with a medium-hold aerosol hair spray for volume and flexible hold.

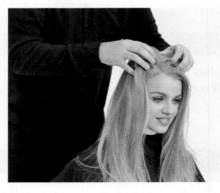

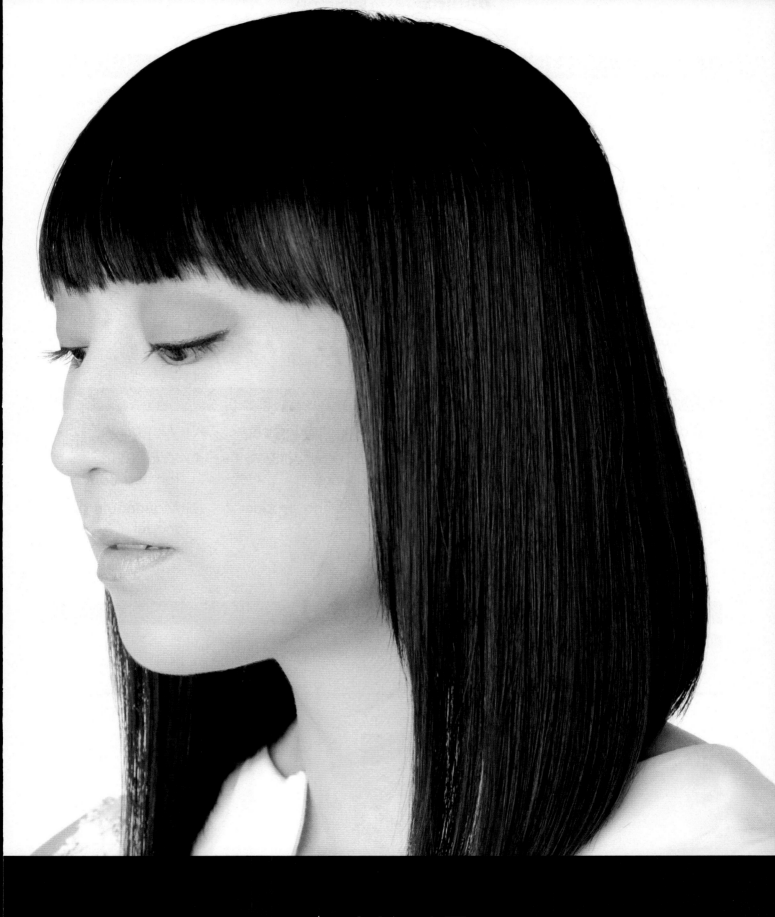

A-LINE

After completing this section, you will be able to **perform** and **diagram** the A-Line haircut. You will also **understand** and be able to **identify** the differences between the A-Line and the Blunt Haircut, as well as how to make the A-Line suitable for all guests.

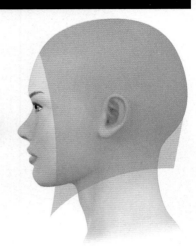

DESCRIPTION

The classic A-Line stems from the Blunt Haircut, with added forward movement that lends the cut its signature shape. While the angles of the lines and partings are steeper in the A-Line, the distribution (natural fall) and elevation (zero degrees) remain the same. The interior can optionally be layered at 90 degrees, ensuring consistency in your one-length line. You will understand how to create the A-Line, how zero degrees of elevation creates a haircut with maximum density, and how diagonal forward section angles help push or distribute weight forward.

MATERIALS AND SUPPLIES

- ☐ Blowdryer
- ☐ Classic styling brush
- ☐ Cutting cape
- ☐ Cutting comb
- ☐ Flat iron
- ☐ Haircutting shears
- ☐ Neck strip
- ☐ Round brush
- ☐ Sectioning clips
- ☐ Spray bottle with water
- ☐ Styling product
- ☐ Towels
- ☐ Vent brush
- ☐ Wide-/Fine-toothed combs
- ☐ Mannequin or model

STEPS TO HAIRCUT

1 Carry out the **Guest Preparation Procedure**.

2 Detangle the hair using a wide-tooth comb.

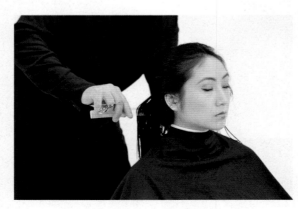

3 Place a center part from the forehead to the nape. Make sure that your lines, sections, and partings are neat and balanced – use your mirror to ensure accuracy.

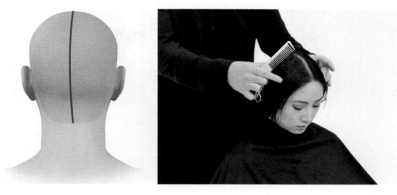

4 Next, create two steep diagonal forward partings from the occipital to the bottom of each ear, then from this section, take a ½-inch (1.3-cm) wide subsection. The depth and width of the section may vary due to hair density.

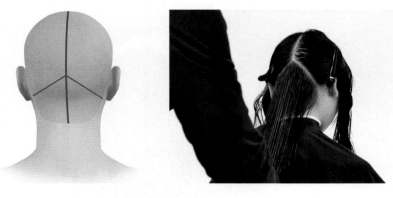

5 Angle the head forward slightly. Begin in the center and, using the fine teeth, comb the hair to its natural fall. Cut your first line parallel to the steep diagonal forward parting, at zero-degree elevation.

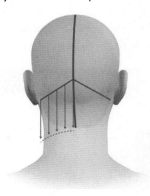
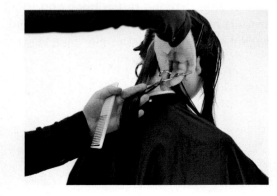

6 Repeat on the opposite side, starting the cut from the outer corner and moving to the center, creating a steep arc shape. Cross-check for balance and to ensure proper length.

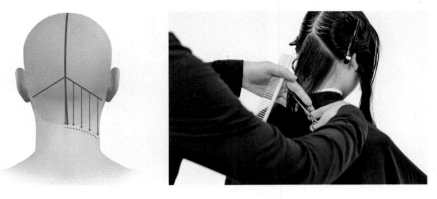

7 Place another set of steep diagonal forward subsections (about an inch [2.5 cm]) from above the occipital to the middle of each ear. The head position will move up slightly, but the natural fall distribution and zero-degree elevation will remain consistent. Cut parallel to the partings and follow the length of your guide from the previously cut section.

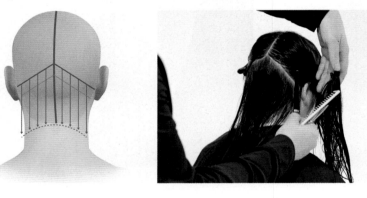

8 Beginning just below the crown, place another set of steep diagonal subsections extending to the low recession on either side. Starting in the back and using the wide teeth, comb the hair over the previously cut hair to its natural fall (zero-degree elevation). Following your guide, cut along the comb until you reach the sides, parallel to the steep diagonal forward parting.

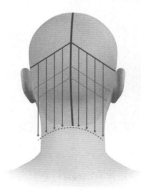
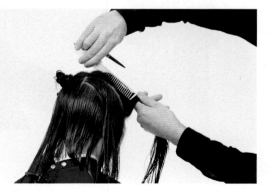

9 Position the guest's head upright. On the sides just behind the ear, continue to comb the hair to natural fall (elevation at zero degrees), cutting the hair parallel to the steep diagonal forward parting. Pay close attention to the protrusion of the ear, and be sure to tap the hair above the comb before you cut to release any tension.

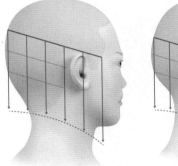 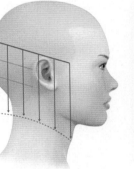 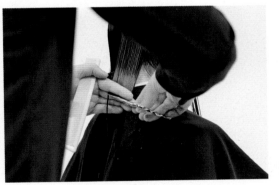

10 Repeat on the opposite side to create balance. Before moving on, stand behind the guest and check that the lengths on both sides are the same length. Make any needed adjustments.

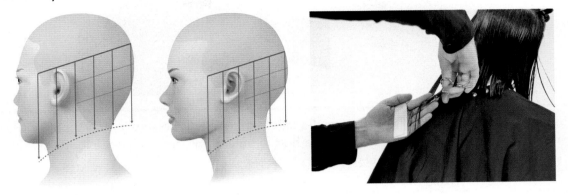

11 When ready, take another set of steep diagonal subsection from above the crown to mid-recession. Starting at the back, comb the hair to natural fall and cut at zero degrees, following your guide. Repeat **Steps 9 and 10** when you reach the sides.

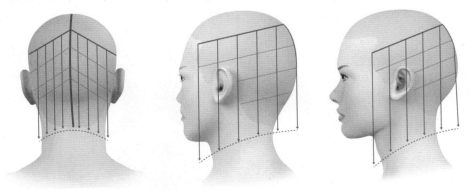

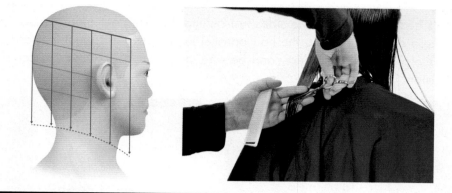

12 Release the remaining hair in the section and comb to natural fall. Be sure to notice any cowlicks or movement at the crown. Continue combing the hair to natural fall, from the back to the sides. Follow your guide and cut at zero-degree elevation.

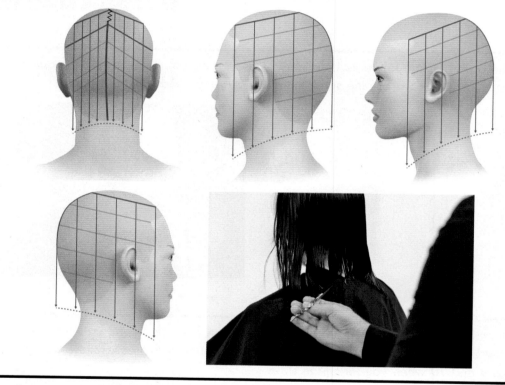

13 Perform a fringe consultation and cut the bangs as desired.

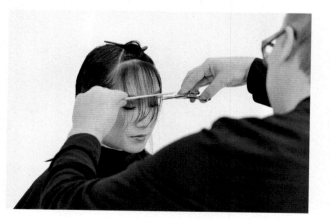

FINISH DESCRIPTION

The A-Line can be applied to different textures of hair; as such, you should adapt your finish to the texture at hand.

FINISH PREPARATION

When working on straight hair, a classic styling brush is recommended. If the guest has curls, the hair can be round brushed or diffused. A flat iron may be required if the hair needs a more polished look. Use products according to the texture. For example, a volumizing mousse works best on fine-to-medium textured hair; gels and creams work best on thick, coarse hair and curls.

STEPS TO FINISH

14 Begin styling by applying a smoothing cream or thermal protectant and working it evenly through the hair.

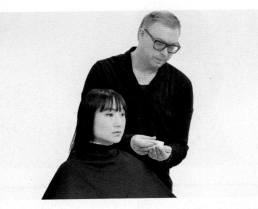

15 To check the line for accuracy, blowdry the hair straight and smooth. Section the hair the same way it was cut, using a classic styling brush if the hair is straight and a round brush if the hair has waves or curls.

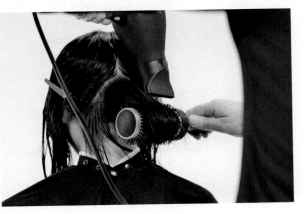

16 Once the haircut is dry, check the line in the mirror. You should see a balanced, steep diagonal forward line going from short at the nape to longer at the sides – the fabled A-line itself.

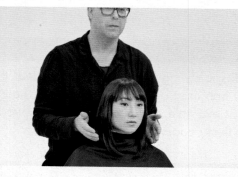

17 Using the wide teeth, comb the hair to natural fall and clean up your one-length line. Avoid cutting your line shorter.

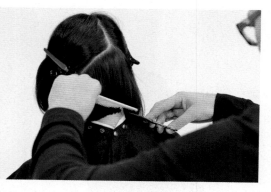

18 To complete the finish, continue blowdrying, using a classic styling brush for straight hair or round brush for curly or wavy hair. A flat iron can be used on dried hair to create a smooth, sleek look.

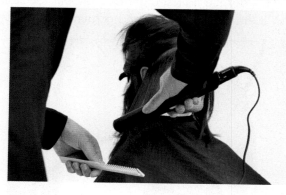

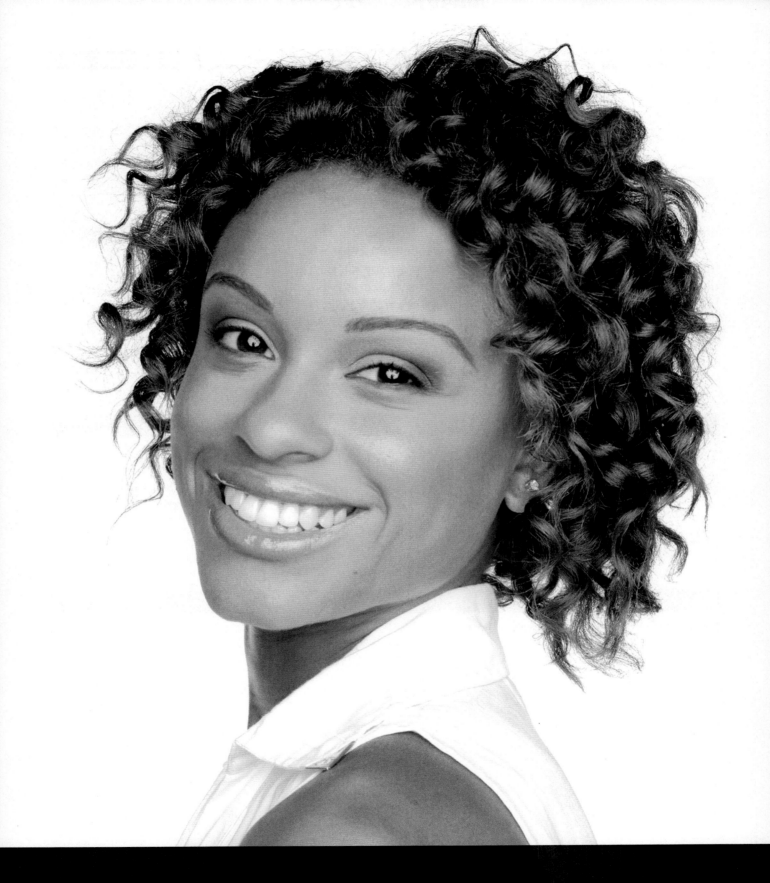

LAYERED BOB

After completing this section, you will be able to **perform** and **diagram** the Layered Bob. You will also **understand** and be able to **identify** the characteristics of the Layered Bob haircut, including why it is layered and what guest would benefit from the layering.

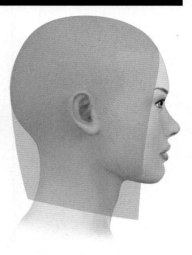

DESCRIPTION

A modern approach to a classic shape. This haircut draws on the techniques and principles of the four foundational haircuts. What separates this particular haircut from others is that it uses elevation to reduce weight in the haircut, whereas a true one-length, one-level, or pageboy all use zero degrees of elevation throughout the entire cut. This haircut is achieved by first establishing the length as done in the Long-Layered Haircut, then moving inward and applying round layers to the interior as shown on shorter hair with the Uniform Layered Haircut. Afterward, the shape is texturized, creating softness and movement while maintaining the bob line. Bangs are optional.

MATERIALS AND SUPPLIES

- ☐ Blowdryer
- ☐ Cutting cape
- ☐ Cutting comb
- ☐ Diffuser
- ☐ Haircutting shears
- ☐ Neck strip
- ☐ Sectioning clips
- ☐ Spray bottle with water
- ☐ Styling product
- ☐ Towels
- ☐ Wide-tooth comb
- ☐ Mannequin or model

STEPS TO HAIRCUT

1. Carry out the **Guest Preparation Procedure**.

2️⃣ Detangle the hair using a wide-tooth comb.

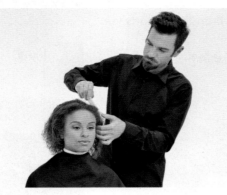

3️⃣ Create a profile section by placing a part from the center of the forehead to the nape. A center parting will allow the guest to wear the style to either side. A side parting is optional.

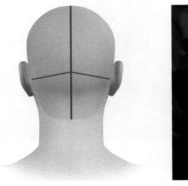
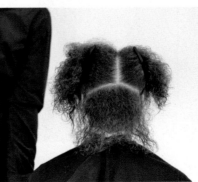

4️⃣ Beginning at the center part, next place two slightly diagonal forward partings extending from the occipital bone to the middle of each ear, creating two large subsections in the area below. Isolate all hair above the occipital, out of the way with clips. Make sure that your lines, sections, and partings are neat and balanced – use your mirror to ensure accuracy.

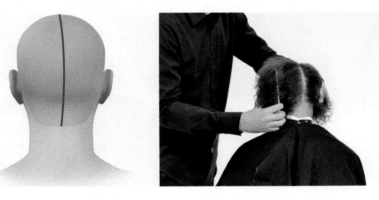

5 Comb the hair to natural fall and angle your fingers parallel to the floor. Standing directly behind the section on your non-dominant side, elevate the section to one-finger depth and cut your line square. Your length should be no longer than the collarbone.

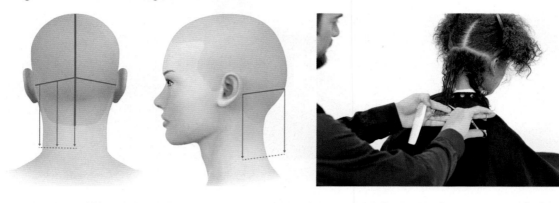

6 Repeat the same technique on the opposite side.

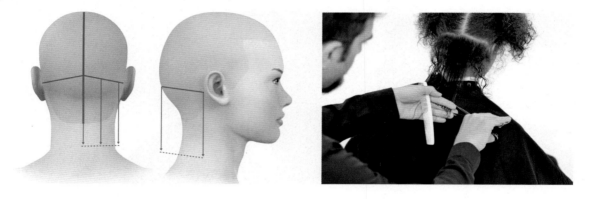

7 Place another set of slight diagonal forward subsection to the top of each ear, elevated to one-finger depth, and cut the line square, following your guide.

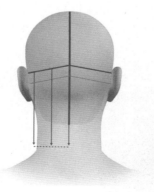
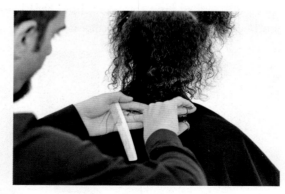

8 Repeat the same technique on the opposite side.

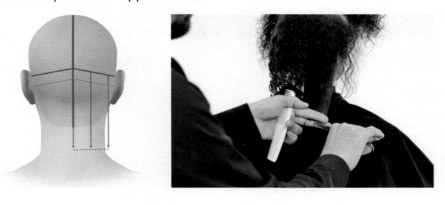

9 Incorporate the sides by placing a horseshoe section from just below the crown to the parietal ridge on both sides. Comb the hair to natural fall and, parallel to your partings, elevate the section to one-finger depth, and cut your line square. When transitioning in to the side, use minimum tension at the ear area and overdirect the hair to the back to retain length. Repeat the same technique on the opposite side.

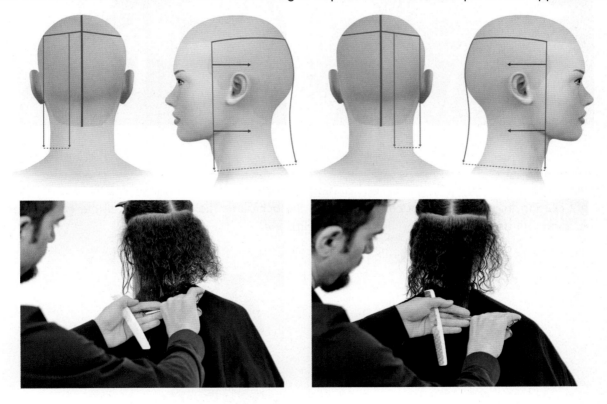

10 Release the remainder of the horseshoe section. Place a parting from the center of the forehead to the crown. Comb the hair to natural fall, elevate the section to one-finger depth, and cut the line square. Following the guide from underneath, complete the sides and the back.

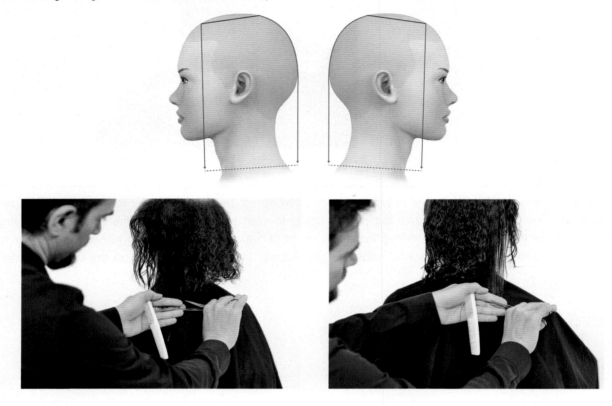

11 Create an arc section by taking a curved parting from the top of each ear across the crown and a straight parting from the top of each ear, through the occipital. The hair in front of the ear and on top of the head will be isolated out of the way with clips.

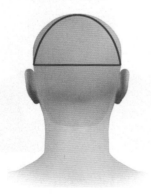
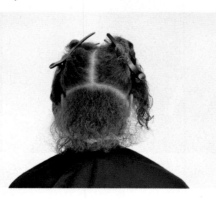

12 At the top of the arc, take a ½-inch (1.3-cm) wide, pivoting or pie-shaped section extending to the occipital. Elevate your section out at 90 degrees and cut your layers with the round of the head, using the length of the hair at the occipital as a guide. To ensure consistency in your cutting line and elevation, subdivide the length of your sections as you work, if necessary.

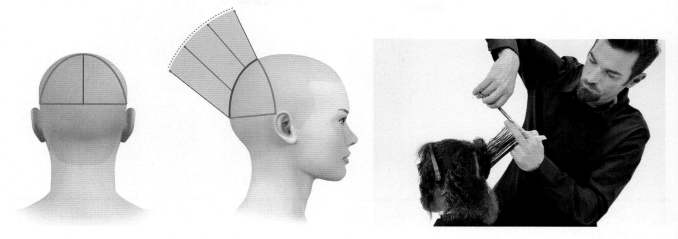

13 Working your way toward the ear, take another ½-inch (1.3-cm) wide, pivoting subsection, elevate the hair out at 90 degrees and cut round, using your previously cut section as a traveling guide.

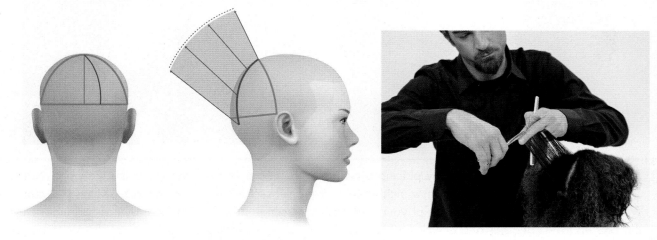

14 Continue taking ½-inch (1.3-cm) wide, pivoting subsections, elevating the hair out at 90 degrees, and cutting with the round of the head. Your line for each cut should follow your guide from the previous section.

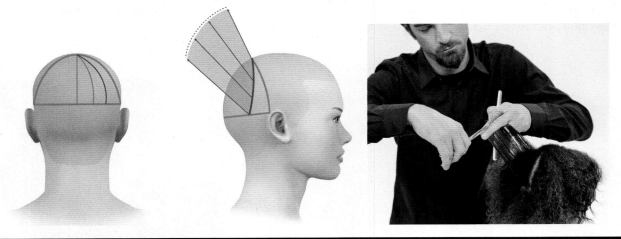

15 Once you have reached the parting at the ear, switch body position and repeat the same technique on the opposite side.

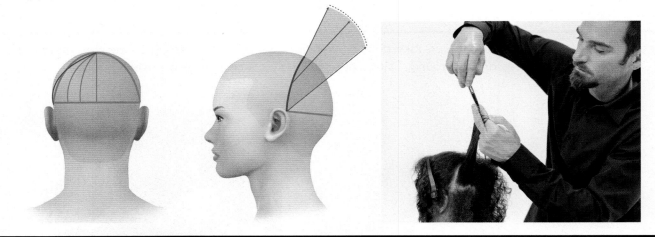

16 At the top, create a band section by placing a part from the center of the forehead to the crown. On either side of the center part, section out a ¼-inch (0.6-cm) wide subsection of hair, creating a ½-inch (1.3-cm) wide band section. Using the length of your previously cut section from behind the crown as a guide, elevate the hair up to 90 degrees and overdirect back to the crown, so your length is going from shorter to longer. Cut parallel to your finger angle.

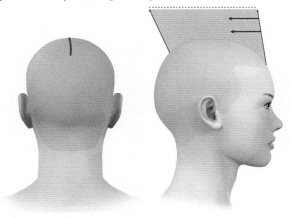

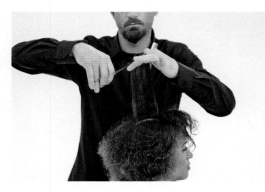

17 Create a parting from the center of the forehead to the crown. Place a diagonal forward parting from the crown to the sideburn in front of the ear. In front of the parting, take a ½-inch (1.3-cm) wide, diagonal forward subsection from the front hairline to the center part. Elevate the hair up to 90 degrees, overdirect back to the length of your previously cut section behind the ear, and cut.

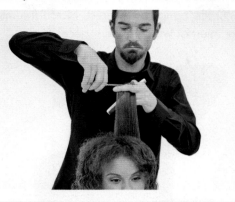

18 Continue taking ½-inch (1.3-cm) wide, diagonal forward subsections, elevating the hair up to 90 degrees, overdirecting back to the previously cut section behind the ear, and cutting. Repeat this technique until you reach the subsection at the front hairline, and then repeat the same technique on the opposite side. When complete, cross-check for balance on both sides.

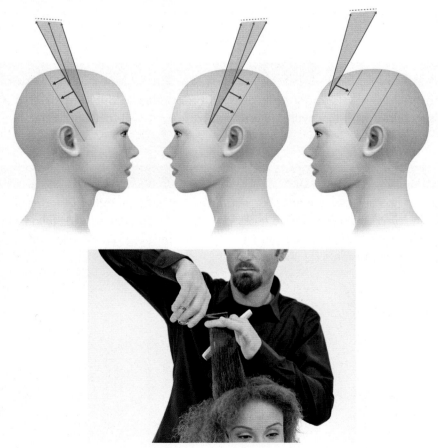

19 If more texture is desired upon completing the cut, go back in once dry and notch into your length at the back and sides, softening your line.

20 Perform a fringe consultation and cut the bangs as desired. Notch the interior to soften and remove weight. Slicing can also be used to remove internal weight where necessary.

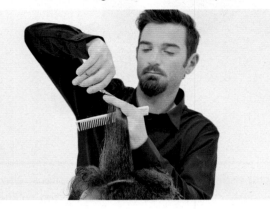

21 Utilize the mirror when detailing your haircut, as you move the hair around to check for balance.

FINISH DESCRIPTION

This haircut works best on wavy to straight hair, but can be applied to different textures of hair. The shape should have a visible textured bob line with textured round layers, with optional bangs.

FINISH PREPARATION

The finish for this haircut has several options. For example, apply a smoothing cream before you blowdry and finish with a serum for a smoother classic look, or a texturizing pomade for fullness, texture, and separation. When finishing any haircut, you must choose the finishing techniques and products that best support your guest's needs and wants for their style.

STEPS TO FINISH

22 Apply a cream thermal protectant, comb through for even distribution. Distribute styling product through slightly wet hair with your fingers and comb through with a wide-tooth comb. Always use products designed for this type of hair texture.

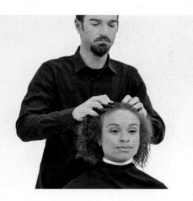

23 Position the hair the way the client likes to wear it. Avoid placing a side part before diffusing; it will leave a line of demarcation. If the client wears it to the side, wait until the hair is 100 percent dry before placing a side part.

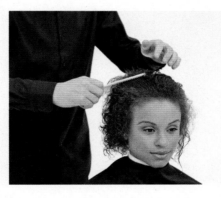

24 Attach the diffuser to the blowdryer and have the client tilt their head back or bend forward. Diffuse the hair by letting the hair sit on top of the diffuser and pulsing the dryer toward the scalp and then away, repeating until the section is dry.

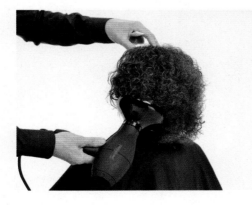

25 Once the hair is completely dry, shake the hair but avoid running your fingers through it or using a comb or brush. Use your fingers to separate the curl if necessary. Finish the haircut with a serum for a smoother look or a wax for texture and separation.

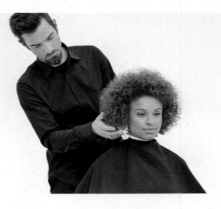

TEXTURED GRADUATION

LEARNING OBJECTIVES

After completing this section, you will be able to **perform** and **diagram** the Textured Graduation. You will also **understand** and be able to **identify** the differences between the Textured Graduation and the Graduated Haircut, as well as how texture is created.

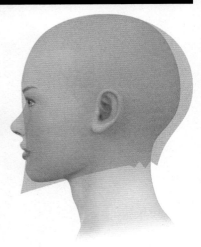

DESCRIPTION

This look is achieved by combining vertical graduation with layering. You will see that Textured Graduation uses similar sectioning and overdirection to that of the Graduated Haircut. However, Textured Graduation incorporates point cutting to create movement and uses a range of elevations to both build and remove weight. The use of point cutting to create texture, softness, and versatility gives this classic style a modern edge. Overdirection also plays a part in creating more length in the front, combined with a stationary guide.

MATERIALS AND SUPPLIES

- ☐ Blowdryer
- ☐ Classic styling brush
- ☐ Cutting cape
- ☐ Cutting comb

- ☐ Flat iron
- ☐ Haircutting shears
- ☐ Neck strip
- ☐ Round brush

- ☐ Sectioning clips
- ☐ Spray bottle with water
- ☐ Styling product
- ☐ Towels

- ☐ Wide-tooth comb
- ☐ Mannequin or model

STEPS TO HAIRCUT

1 Carry out the **Guest Preparation Procedure**.

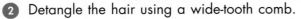

2 Detangle the hair using a wide-tooth comb.

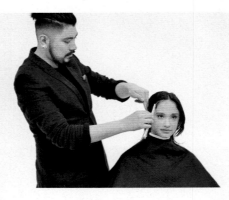

3 Place a horseshoe section from just below the crown to the parietal ridge on both sides. At the back, place a center parting extending from the bottom of the horseshoe through the nape. Then, place a diagonal forward parting from the horseshoe to just behind each ear. Make sure that your section and partings are neat and balanced – use the mirror to ensure accuracy. Isolate all hair above the horseshoe and in front of the ears out of the way in clips.

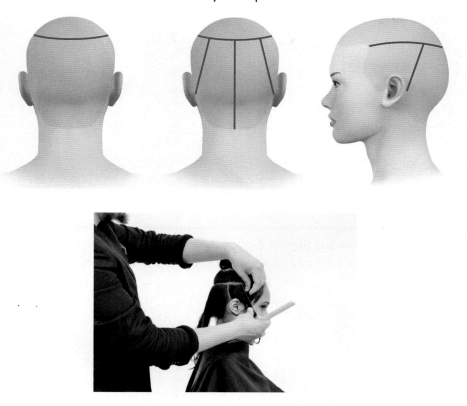

4 Next, starting to the left of the center part, take a ½-inch (1.3-cm) wide, slightly diagonal forward subsection, extending from the bottom of the horseshoe through the nape. Isolate all hair to either side of the subsection out of the way.

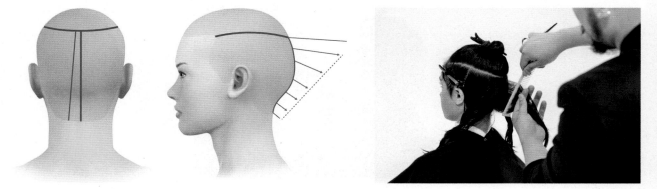

5 For control and easier handling, you will subdivide the subsection, holding in your hand only enough hair that you are able to cut, to the left of the center part. Beginning at the top of your subsection, comb the hair out at 90 degrees from the head, angle your fingers at 45 degrees, then cut your graduation approximately 4 inches (10.2 cm) in length, decreasing to 3 inches (7.6 cm) at the nape – your finger angle will create the vertical graduation.

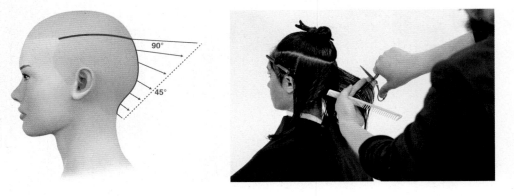

6 Take another ½-inch (1.3-cm) wide, slightly diagonal forward subsection. Comb the hair out from the head at 90 degrees, angle your fingers at 45 degrees, and cut your line, traveling with the guide from the previously cut section.

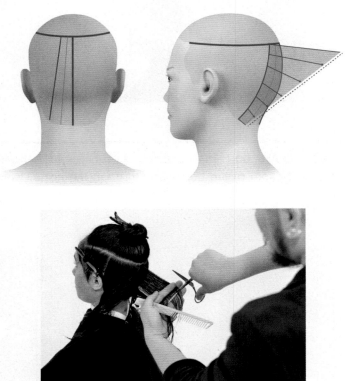

7 Proceed with this technique until you reach the parting behind the ear. Next, starting on the right side of the center part, repeat the same technique on the opposite side. Your hand position will now change: reverse your hand and cut palm to palm with fingers facing down. Keeping the elbow up on your non-cutting hand will ensure consistency with the graduation.

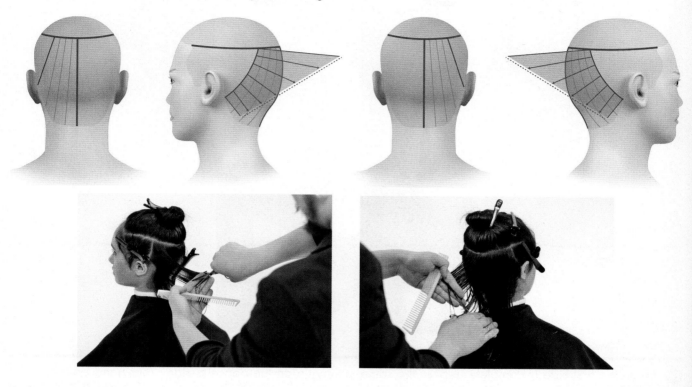

8 Check for balance once you have completed the back. Resume at the diagonal forward part behind the left ear. At this point, your guide will change from traveling to stationary in order to maintain more length. Take a ½-inch (1.3-cm) wide, diagonal forward subsection from the horseshoe section to the middle of the ear. Overdirect the subsection back to your guide behind the ear, and cut your line.

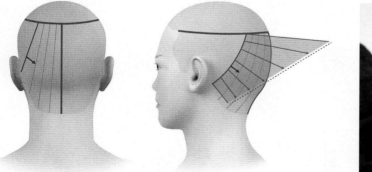
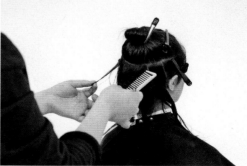

9 Continue taking ½-inch (1.3-cm) wide, diagonal forward subsections, overdirecting them back and cutting to the stationary guide behind the ear. Repeat this technique until you complete the side.

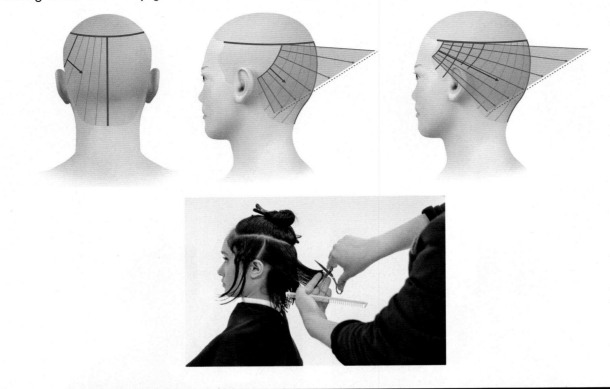

10 Once the first side is complete, repeat the same technique on the opposite side. Your hand position will change again: reverse your hand and cut palm to palm with fingers facing down. Check for balance.

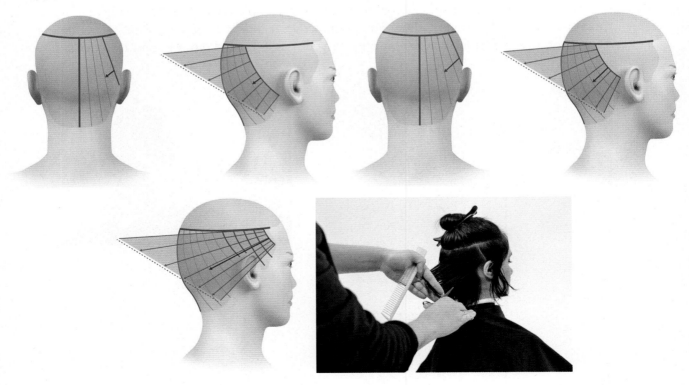

11 When the graduation is complete comb the hair around the perimeter down and, if needed, detail the length by point cutting at the nape and sides to create a soft textured line.

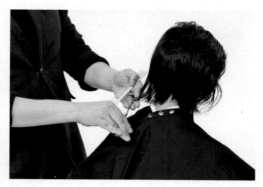

12 Release the top horseshoe section and create an arc section by taking a curved parting from the top of each ear across the crown, and then from the top of each ear through the occipital. Isolate all hair in front of the ear out of the way with clips. Once the hair in the arc has been sectioned, place a center parting from the center of the forehead to the crown.

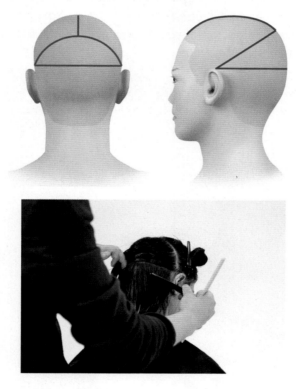

13 At the top of the arc, take a ½-inch (1.3-cm) wide, pivoting subsection to the occipital and elevate the section out from the head at 90 degrees, revealing the top of the graduation. Using the top of the graduation as a guide point, cut with the round of the head and connect the top of the graduation to the hair in the crown.

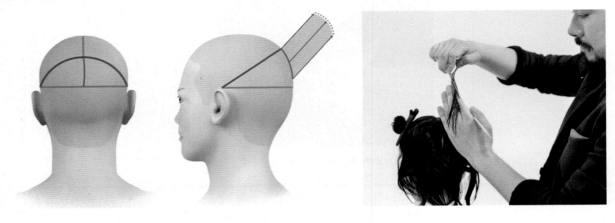

14 Continue to take ½-inch (1.3-cm) wide, pivoting sections, elevated to 90 degrees, cutting round and working your way from the center part out to the left ear. Follow your guide from the previously cut section and make sure you begin cutting your line from the top of your graduation. Follow this technique until you have reached the curved parting at the top of the ear.

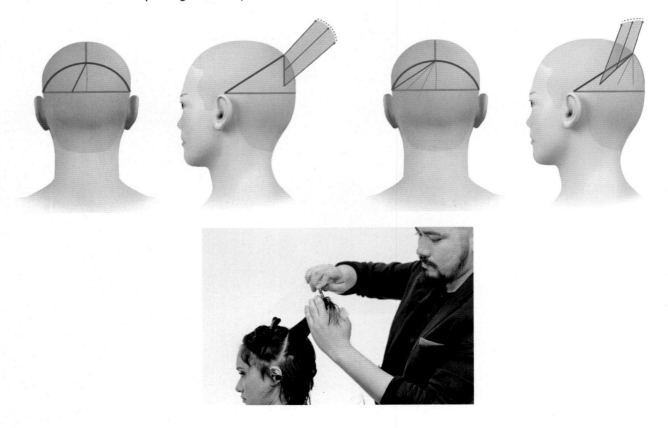

15 Repeat the same technique on the opposite side of the arc section.

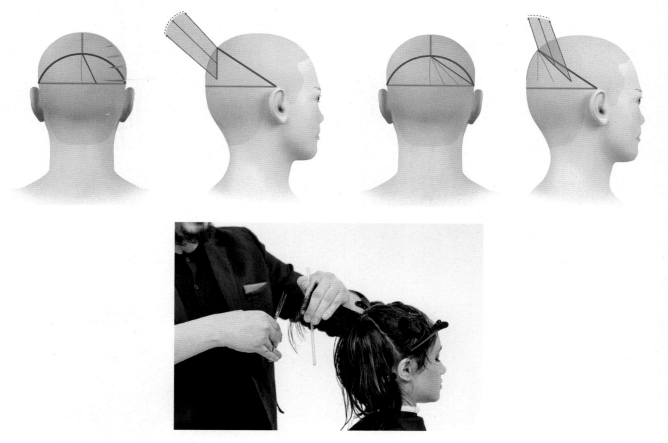

16 Begin your layering for the top of the head at the parietal ridge by taking a ½-inch (1.3-cm) wide, diagonal forward pivoting section, from the crown to the front of the ear. Elevate up to 90 degrees, overdirect back to your previously cut section in the crown, and cut your line.

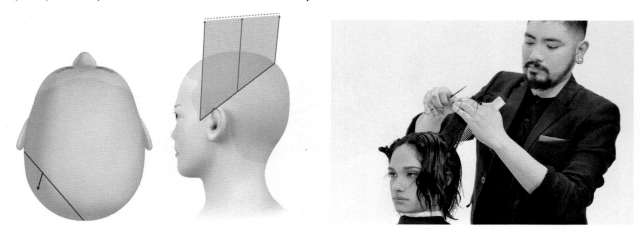

17 Continue taking ½-inch (1.3-cm) wide, diagonal forward pivoting sections, elevating the hair up to 90 degrees, overdirecting them back to your previously cut section, and cutting round layers until you reach the center part. Once you have completed the first side, switch body position and repeat the same technique on the opposite side.

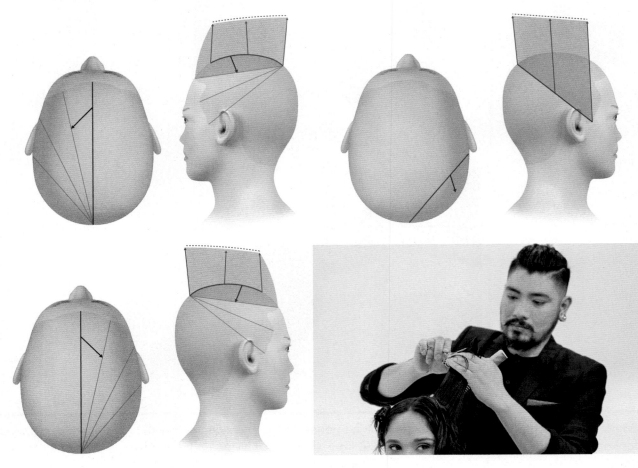

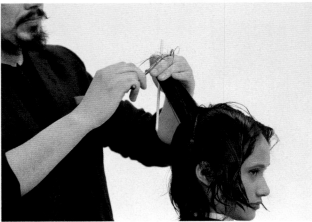

18 Cross-check the top of the cut by taking horizontal sections. You will notice a slight point at the center of the line – point cut to soften this corner and ensure balance. The rest of the haircut will be completed when the hair has been blowdried.

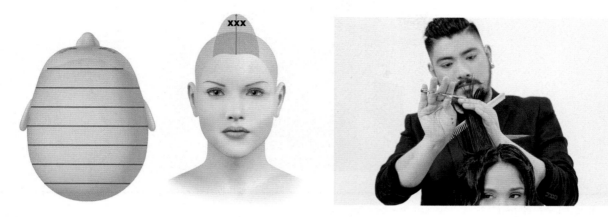

19 If more texture is desired, detail the perimeter by utilizing point cutting. This technique will allow more control when removing excess weight and softening your line.

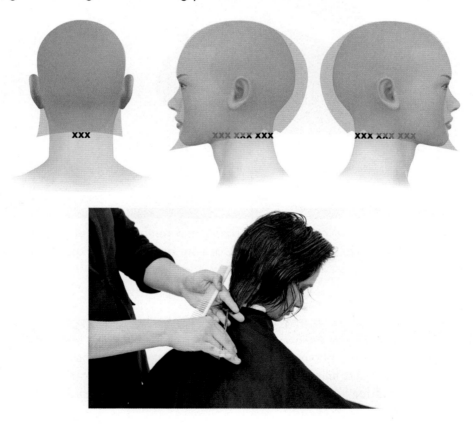

20 Texturize the interior of the haircut with notching. If you need to remove weight internally, use slicing to create movement and volume.

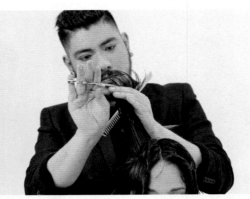

21 Perform a fringe consultation and cut the bangs if desired.

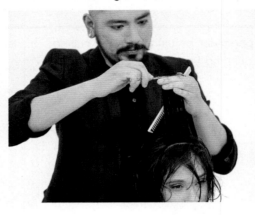

FINISH DESCRIPTION

This shape should have versatility built into it. By texturizing and removing the proper amount of weight, the haircut can be worn straight, smooth, and conservative, or with an edge, by exposing the texturizing with product.

FINISH PREPARATION

The finish for this haircut has several options, depending on the texture of the hair. Smoothing cream, light gel, or mousse can give softness and fullness. Alternatively, apply a serum for a smoother classic look, or a light wax or texturizing pomade for fullness, texture, and separation. If you desire a sleeker look, finish with a flat iron.

22 Apply a medium-hold mousse and a thermal protectant, and comb through for even distribution. Starting on the sides, section the hair into 2-inch (5.1-cm) panels and begin blowdrying with either a classic styling brush or round brush. The hair should be straight and smooth when completed – blowdrying in a forward direction helps to create smoothness.

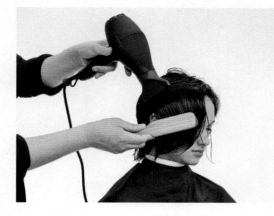

23 Flat iron the hair if necessary.

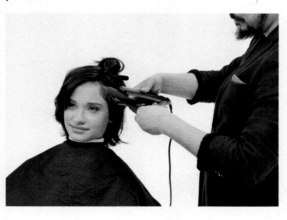

24 Finish the look by applying a light wax or texturizing pomade. This will achieve volume, texture, and separation.

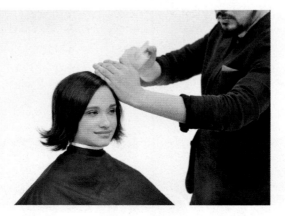

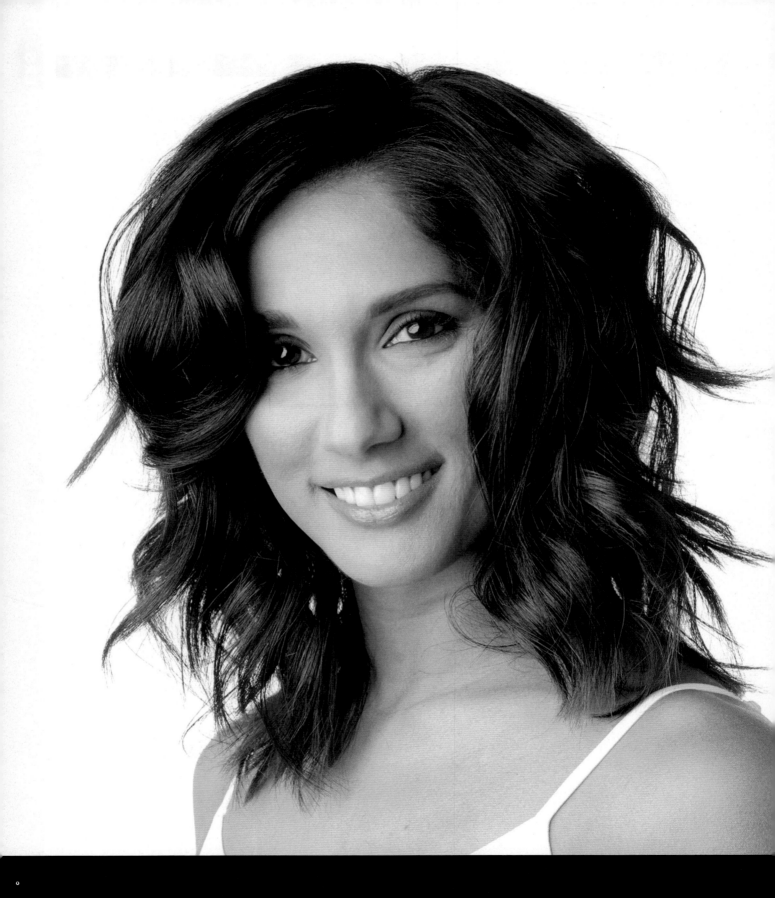

MID-LENGTH LAYERS

LEARNING OBJECTIVES

After completing this section, you will be able to **perform** and **diagram** the Mid-Length Layers haircut. You will also **understand** and be able to **identify** mid-length layers, what makes them mid-length, and why they are so versatile.

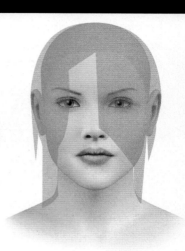

DESCRIPTION

This haircut is ideal for shoulder- to collarbone-length hair. Mid-Length Layers is similar to the Uniform Layered Haircut, as it creates a uniform length in the back by using a traveling guide, and everything is cut at 90 degrees of elevation. However, because the top is cut using a stationary guide combined with overdirection, Mid-Length Layers is able to preserve length and ensure versatility in styling. Point cutting within the interior layers adds further movement and versatility to the result. Upon completion of this haircut, you will be able to understand and use a combination of overdirections to create haircuts with more versatility, as well as identify and blend the disconnection between two distinct layers.

MATERIALS AND SUPPLIES

- ☐ Blowdryer
- ☐ Cutting cape
- ☐ Cutting comb
- ☐ Flat iron
- ☐ Haircutting shears
- ☐ Neck strip
- ☐ Round brush
- ☐ Sectioning clips
- ☐ Spray bottle with water
- ☐ Styling product
- ☐ Towels
- ☐ Wide-tooth comb
- ☐ Mannequin or model

STEPS TO HAIRCUT

1 Carry out the **Guest Preparation Procedure**.

2 Detangle the hair using a wide-tooth comb.

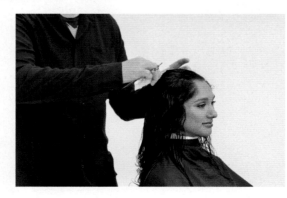

3 Begin by placing a horseshoe section from just below the crown to the parietal ridge on both sides. Isolate the hair above the horseshoe with a sectioning clip. Next, place a diagonal forward parting from the horseshoe to right behind the ear on each side. Make sure that your lines, sections, and partings are neat and balanced – use the mirror to ensure accuracy.

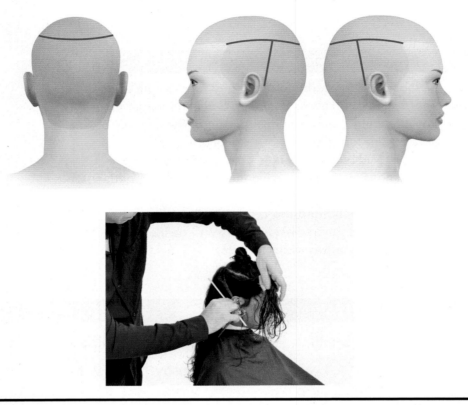

4 Isolate the hair above the horseshoe and in front of the ear with sectioning clips, then take a ½-inch (1.3-cm) wide section from just below the crown to the nape. Comb the hair straight out at 90 degrees from the head and cut your layers square, 10 to 11 inches (25.4 to 27.9 cm) in length.

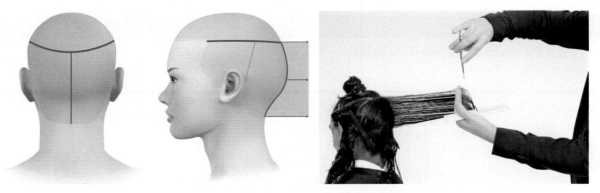

5. Place another ½-inch (1.3-cm) wide, vertical subsection from just below the crown to the nape. Elevate the hair straight out at 90 degrees and cut square, using your previously cut section as a guide. To ensure consistency in your cutting line and elevation, subdivide the length of your sections as you work, if necessary.

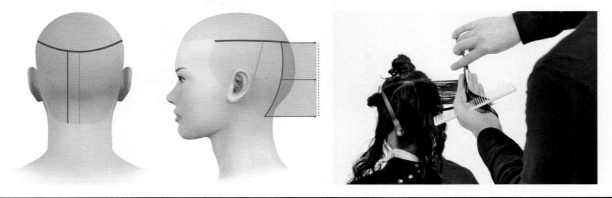

6. Continue taking ½-inch (1.3-cm) wide, vertical subsections, elevating the hair straight out at 90 degrees from the head, using the traveling guide from the previously cut section, and cutting square, until you reach the parting at the ear.

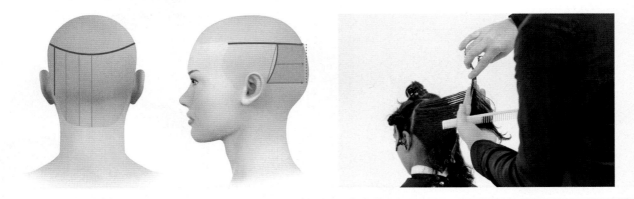

7. Once there, switch body position and repeat the same technique on the opposite side in back, stopping at the parting behind the ear. Cross-check for balance and make any adjustments necessary before moving on to the sides.

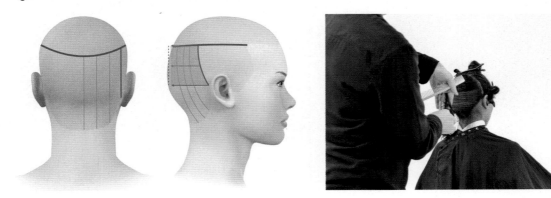

8 When the cross-check is complete, switch body positions again and resume on the side where you started. At the ear, past the round of the head, your subsections will change from vertical to diagonal forward and be overdirected back to the previously cut section.

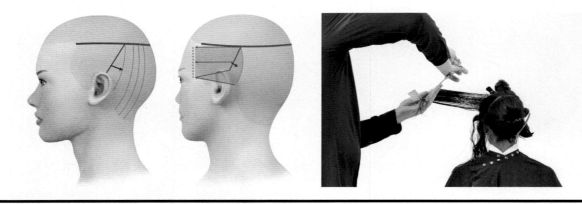

9 In front of the parting, take ½-inch (1.3-cm) wide, diagonal forward subsections, elevate the hair straight out at 90 degrees from the head, overdirect back, and cut your layers square, following your guide from the previously cut section behind the ear.

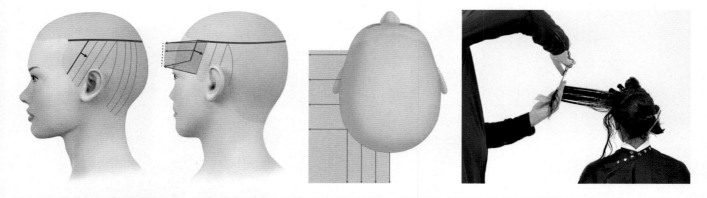

10 Once you have completed one side, switch body positions and repeat the same technique on the opposite side. Check for balance as you move forward with your sections.

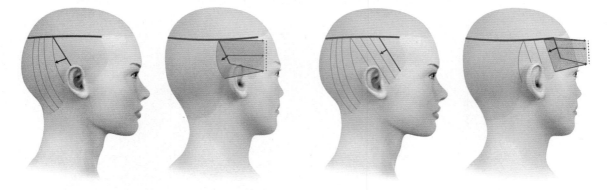

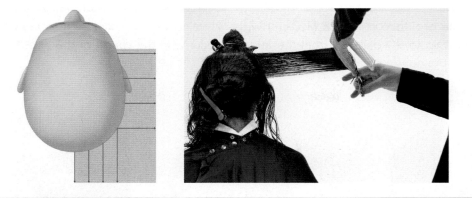

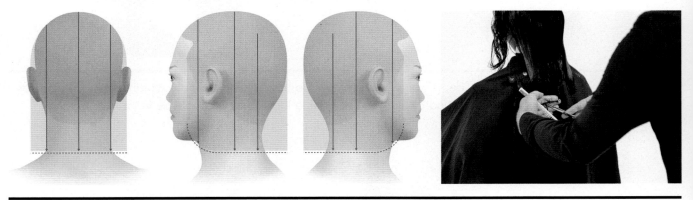

11 After you have completed the back and sides, comb the hair underneath to natural fall and cut square at the back, rounding up toward the jaw as you transition to the sides in front of the ear.

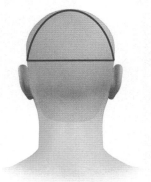
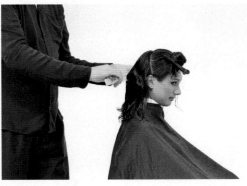

12 Release the top section and place an arc section, by taking a curved parting from the top of each ear across the crown, and a straight parting from the top of each ear through the occipital. Secure all hair above the arc and in front of the ear out of the way with clips.

13 At the top of the arc, take a ½-inch (1.3-cm) wide, pivoting section extending to the occipital. Elevate the hair straight up to 90 degrees from the head and cut with the round of the head, following your guide from the previously cut section below.

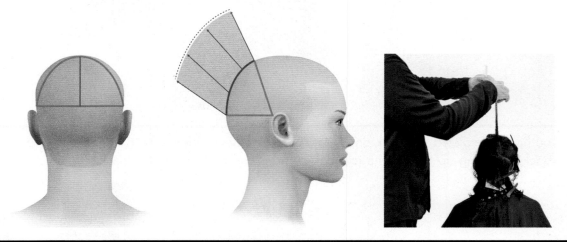

14 Take another ½-inch (1.3-cm) wide, pivoting section from the arc, elevate the hair straight up to 90 degrees from the head, and cut with the round of the head. Continue this technique until you have reached the curved parting at the top of the ear.

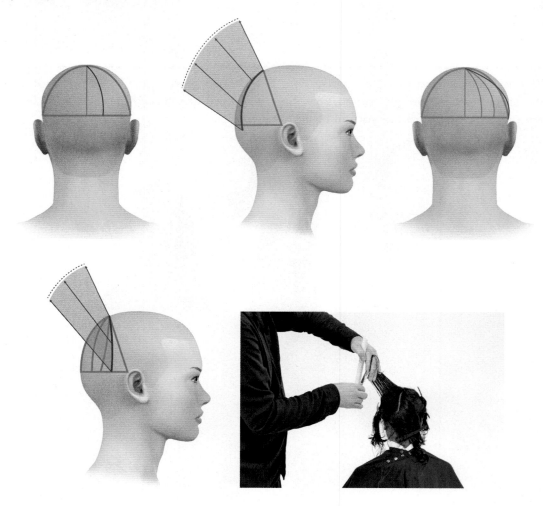

15 Switch body position and repeat on the opposite side of the arc. Before moving on to the top, cross-check for balance.

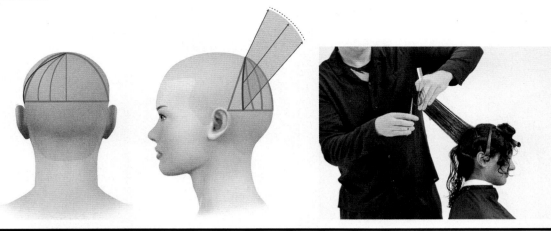

16 The hair at the top will be cut in an asymmetric manner, giving a light and a heavy side to the part over the eye. At the top, create a stationary guide by placing a ½-inch (1.3-cm) wide, pivoting section diagonally from the crown to the corner of one eye. Using the length of your crown as a guide, elevate the hair straight up to 90 degrees from the head and cut your layers square – approximately 8 to 9 inches (20.3 to 22.9 cm) in length – from the crown to the corner of the eye. Note that here there will be a disconnection in length between the crown and parietal ridge.

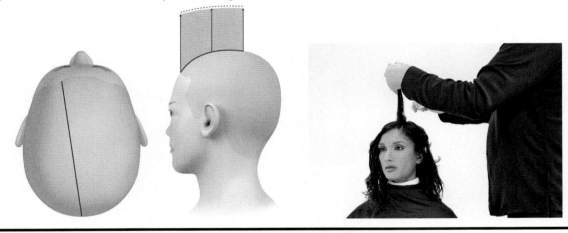

17 Working your way across the top of the heavy side of the part, place another ½-inch (1.3-cm) wide, pivoting section from the crown to the opposite side of the stationary guide. Elevate the hair straight up to 90 degrees from the head, overdirect the section to the stationary guide, and cut.

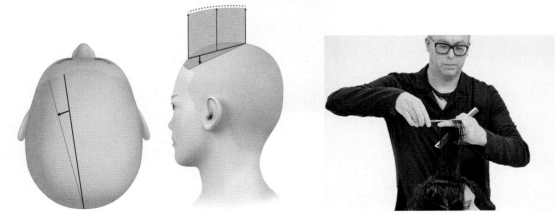

18 Continue taking ½-inch (1.3-cm) wide, pivoting diagonal sections, elevating the hair straight up to 90 degrees from the head, overdirecting to the stationary guide, and cutting. Repeat this technique until you have completed the hair on the heavy side.

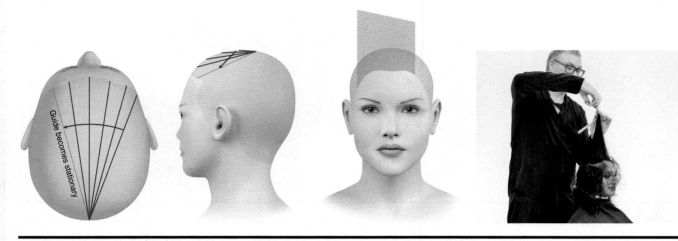

19 Remaining in the same body position, place another ½-inch (1.3-cm) wide, pivoting subsection from the crown to the light side of the stationary guide. Elevate the hair up to 90 degrees, overdirect to the stationary guide, and cut your line square. Repeat until you have completed the section on the side.

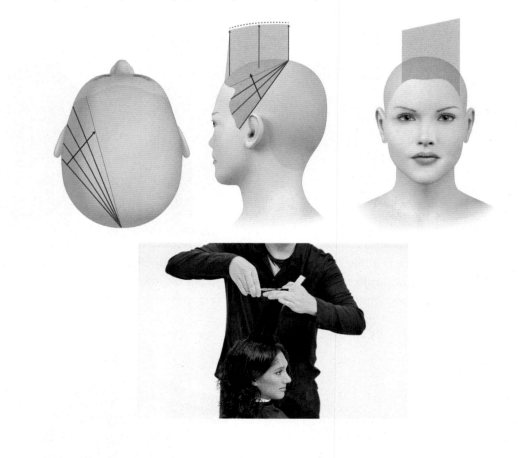

20 Next you will work between the crown and parietal ridge to blend or shatter the disconnection of the top and sides. To do this, you will start by taking a vertical parting from the crown to the parietal ridge. In front of the parting, take a ½-inch (1.3-cm) horizontal subsection, elevate the hair straight out at 90 degrees, overdirect back to the previously cut section in the crown to reveal the disconnection, and use point cutting to blend the weight line.

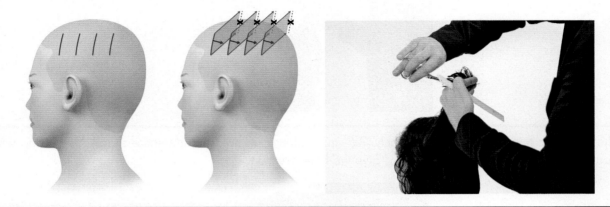

21 Continue taking vertical subsections from the top to the parietal ridge, elevating the sections up to 90 degrees, overdirecting back to the previous cut section, and point cutting to blend your disconnection. Continue this technique until you complete the side.

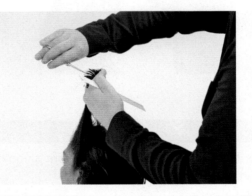

22 Switch body position and repeat the same technique on the opposite side.

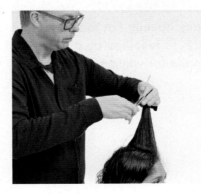

23 If further texture is desired once the hair is dry, detail the length and the perimeter with point cutting.

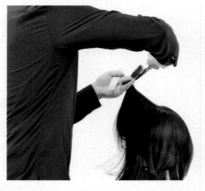

24 The interior is texturized by taking 1-inch (2.5-cm) sections and notching the entire shape. Use slicing when you need to remove excess weight and give the hair direction.

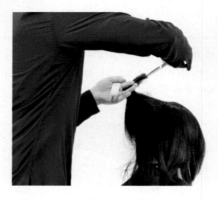

FINISH DESCRIPTION

This shape has a lived-in look to it; however, it can also be worn smooth and straight. Texturizing allows the shape to have movement and versatility.

FINISH PREPARATION

Applying the right products will enhance any haircut. For this shape, we use a light gel for body and a thermal protectant for shine. Use a round brush followed by a flat iron to create a straight and smooth texture. Finish with wax or texturizing pomade for volume and to expose the separation and movement.

25 Apply a light gel and a thermal protectant, and comb through for even distribution. Blowdry the hair using a round brush for volume and texture.

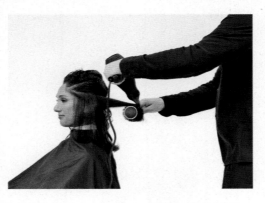

26 Once completely dry, take ½-inch (1.3-cm) panels and flat iron the hair. Finish by applying a wax or texturizing pomade for separation, volume, and movement.

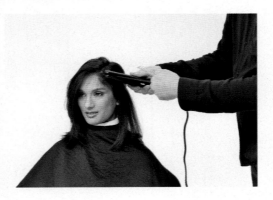

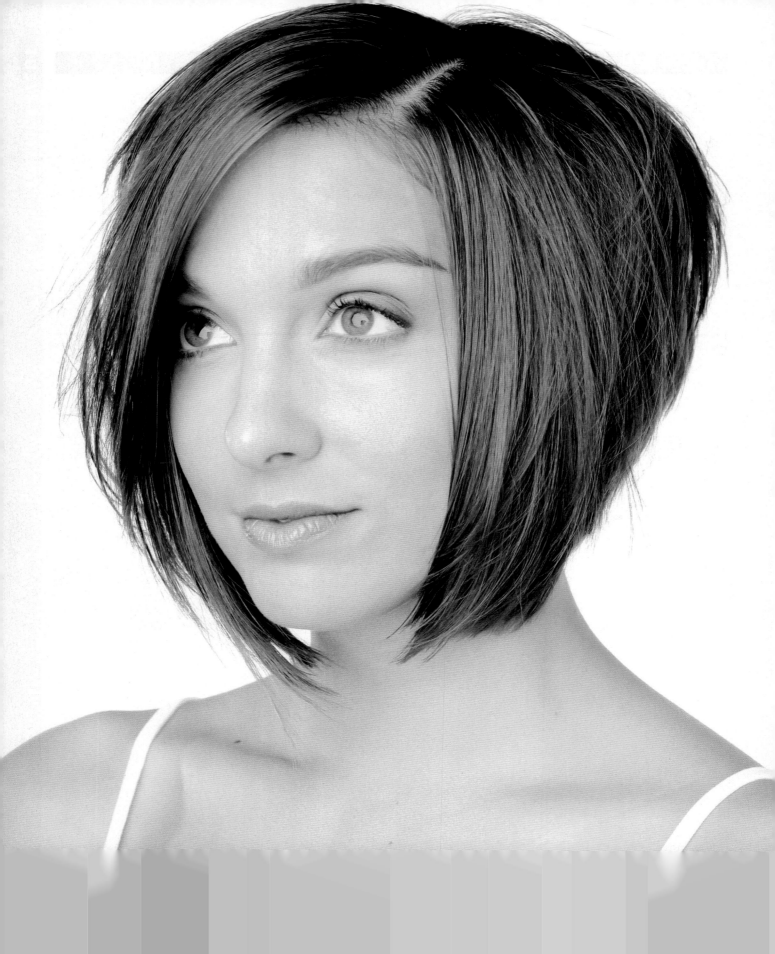

LEARNING OBJECTIVES

After completing this section, you will be able to **perform** and **diagram** the Graduated Haircut. You will also **understand** and be able to **identify** the different levels of graduation that can be created and which one best suits your guest.

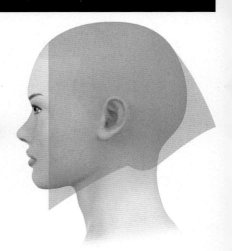

DESCRIPTION

The Graduated Haircut is a modern classic. The sculpted graduation at the nape falls into a beautifully defined weight area at the sides. In this basic haircut, you will be utilizing vertical, horizontal, and diagonal cutting lines with a 45-degree elevation at the back, one-finger depth on the sides, and 90-degree elevation for the layers. Although you will use a side part, keep in mind that this haircut can also work with a center part or a fringe. You will be using a stationary guideline and a traveling guideline – remember, a stationary guideline is a guideline that does not move. All other sections are combed toward the guideline and are cut to match it. A traveling guideline moves with you as you work through the haircut.

MATERIALS AND SUPPLIES

- ☐ Blowdryer
- ☐ Classic styling brush
- ☐ Cutting cape
- ☐ Cutting comb
- ☐ Haircutting shears
- ☐ Neck strip
- ☐ Round brush
- ☐ Sectioning clips
- ☐ Spray bottle with water
- ☐ Styling product
- ☐ Towels
- ☐ Wide-tooth comb
- ☐ Mannequin or model

STEPS TO HAIRCUT

1 Carry out the **Guest Preparation Procedure**.

2 Detangle the hair using a wide-tooth comb.

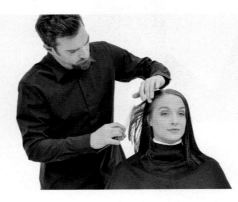

③ Begin your first section by taking the parting from the guest's natural side part back to the crown. Then take a central parting from the crown to the nape. Make sure that your lines, sections, and partings are neat and balanced – use the mirror to ensure accuracy.

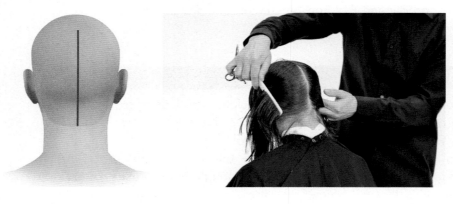

④ At the occipital bone, take a diagonal forward parting from the central parting to the middle of each ear. Then take a ½-inch (1.3-cm) wide, pivoting diagonal forward subsection and elevate it to 45 degrees and cut parallel to your parting. Both your finger angle and elevation should be at 45 degrees.

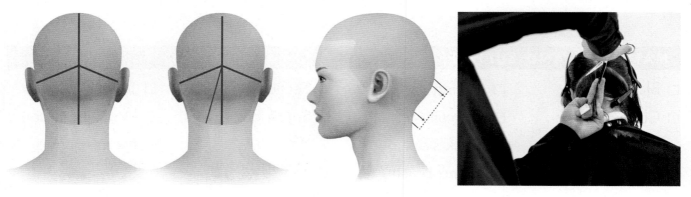

⑤ Make sure that your section is no longer than 2 to 3 inches (5.1 to 7.6 cm) in length or your graduation will sit too low. This will serve as your traveling guide.

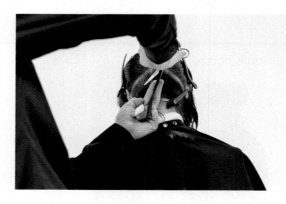

6 Continue taking ½-inch (1.3-cm) wide pivoting diagonal forward subsections, using the previously cut subsection as a traveling guide. Both your elevation and finger angle are held at 45 degrees. Elevate and cut parallel to your parting.

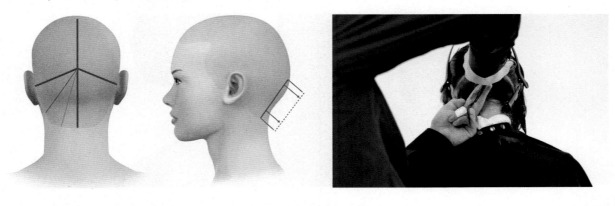

7 Once you have reached your last subsection, you should be parallel to your diagonal forward parting; continue to elevate at 45 degrees, following your traveling guide. Cross-check your section for balance before moving on to the other side.

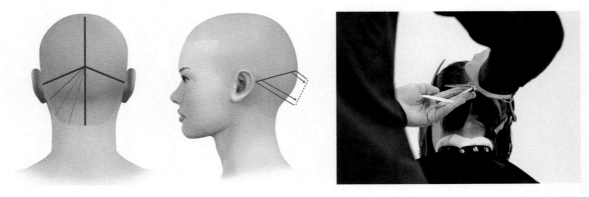

8 Repeat the same steps and technique on the opposite side. Once completed, cross-check the balance from the outer edges on both sides. Clean up any hair left in the perimeter of the nape.

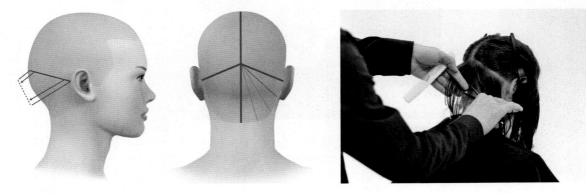

9 To begin the next section, take a diagonal forward parting from above the occipital bone extending to the top of each ear. Each side is then subsectioned and cut as before, using ½-inch (1.3-cm) wide pivoting diagonal forward subsections to work your way through the section.

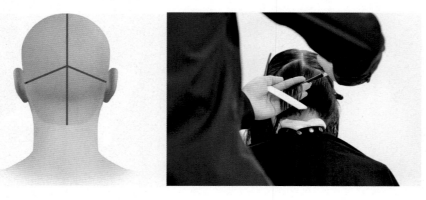

10 To maintain the same level of graduation as the first section, comb the hair parallel to your parting and, using a small piece of the length of hair cut from the last section as a guide, cut a stationary guide at a 45-degree elevation.

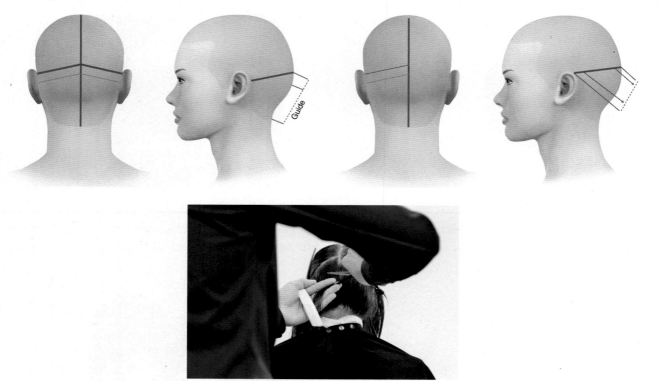

11 Repeat the same steps on the opposite side. Once completed, check for visual balance.

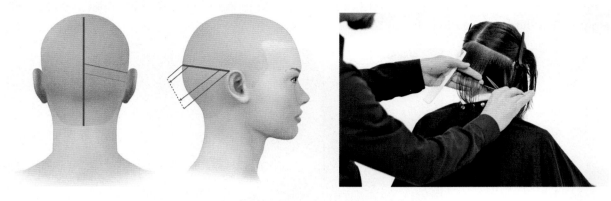

12 The next section will be a horseshoe section taken from just below the crown to the recession area on both sides. Working below the horseshoe, this section will be subdivided and cut using ½-inch (1.3-cm) wide traveling diagonal forward subsections combed to natural fall and then elevated to 45 degrees and cut parallel to the horseshoe parting.

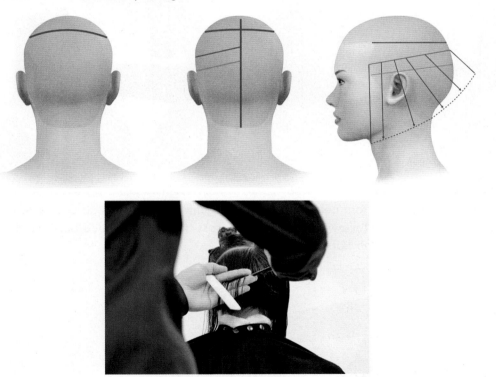

13 The elevation will decrease to one-finger depth just behind the ear where you transition to the sides and the bob line begins. From the ear forward, the hair is held in the fingers at a low elevation to maintain weight within the front hairline.

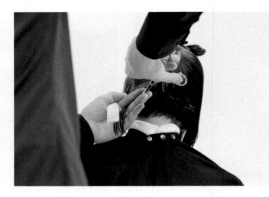

14 Repeat the same steps below the horseshoe on the opposite side.

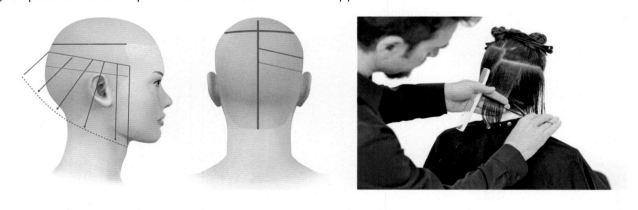

15 Continue taking subsections from below the horseshoe until the natural side part is reached and all remaining hair has been cut following your guide. Cross-check for balance between the left and right sides before moving above the horseshoe.

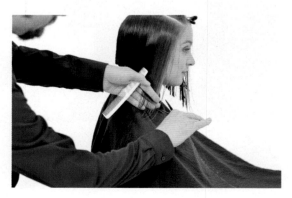

16 To cut the top, you will return to the original side but now above the horseshoe, using the same elevation and cutting technique as before until you reach the guest's natural side part. Repeat this technique on the opposite side.

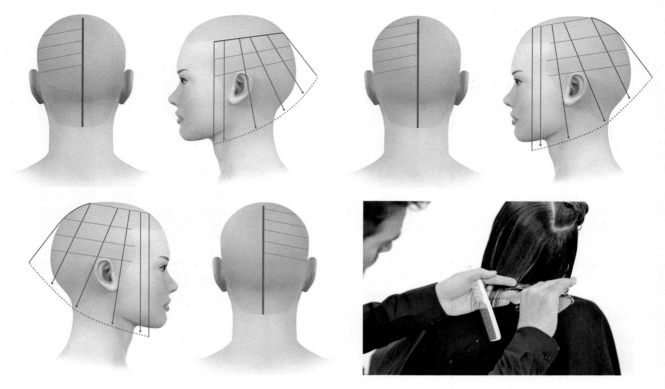

17 In preparation for layering, create a radial section by taking a radial parting from the crown to the top of each ear. Take a ½-inch (1.3-cm) wide, central vertical subsection from the crown to the occipital.

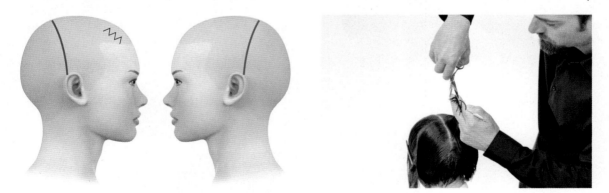

18 The hair in this section is elevated to 90 degrees and, using a traveling guide, overdirected back to your previous section. Your guide will be taken from the perimeter of the graduation for the length. Cut following the head shape. The length will be blended when dry, as the perimeter is detailed.

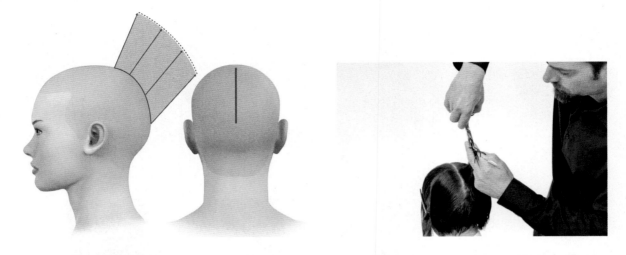

19 One half inch (1.3-cm) wide pivoting subsections are combed to 90 degrees, overdirected back to your previous section and cut parallel to the head. When you have completed the radial section, repeat on the opposite side.

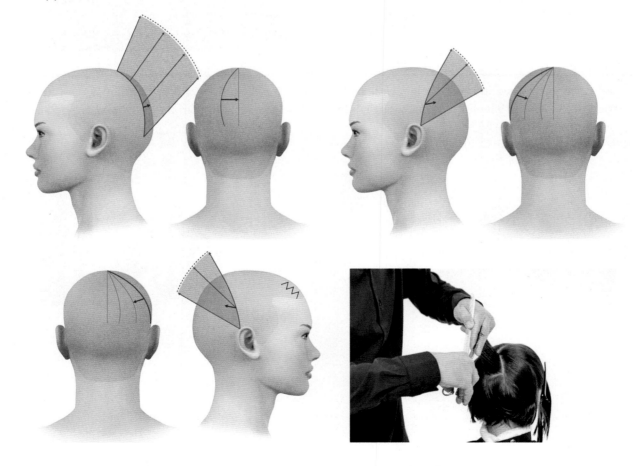

20 When you reach the sides, take a ½-inch (1.3 cm) wide horizontal subsection from the natural side part, elevate to 90 degrees, overdirect back, and cut following your guide from the radial section.

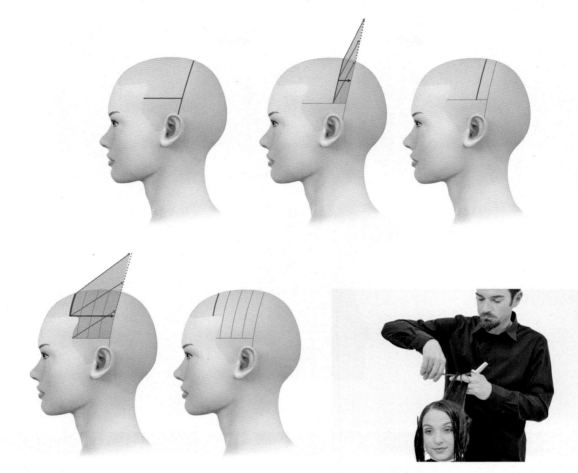

21 In the front, length is maintained by overdirecting back to a stationary guide at the radial section.

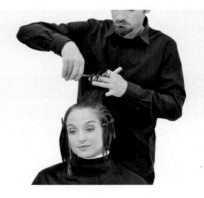

22 Repeat the same steps on the opposite side.

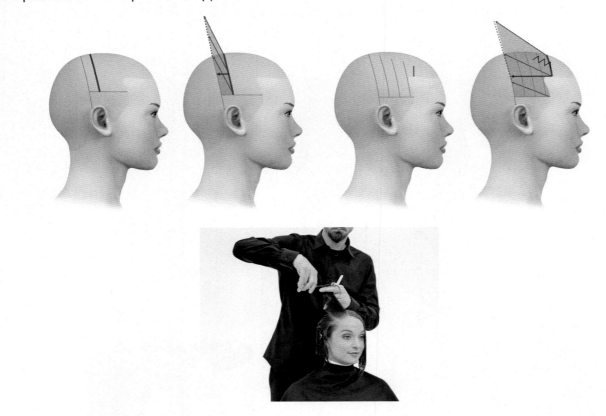

FINISH DESCRIPTION

This graduated haircut is modern in its silhouette, and its diagonal forward line gives great freedom of movement. The close-fitting nape area is very sculptural in nature, while the rest of the cut features great structure and shape. Styling this cut with an asymmetric look is slimming to the face and answers the needs of the guest who wants to wear a side part. The simple movement of the brush and blowdryer through the hair creates body and ornamental effects without diminishing the sculptural silhouette of the cut.

FINISH PREPARATION

To bring the most out of this shape, use a classic styling or paddle brush for smoothness. For a sleek look, follow your blowdry with a flatiron. Add texture to the finish by using a wax or texturizing pomade, to accent pieces in the front or nape area.

23 Apply a thermal protectant and light weight foam and comb through for even distribution. Comb the hair into the desired shape, using the natural side parting.

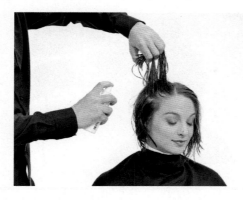

24 Begin blowdrying in the nape area using a classic styling brush followed by a round brush. Flow the hair directionally outward from the center back on either side. The airflow follows the brush as it closely contours the hair against the head.

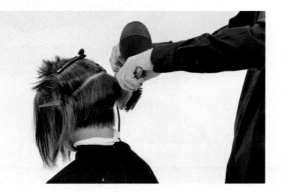

25 Above the occipital area, begin parting out along a diagonal forward line. Continue upward, using the brush while blowdrying along the diagonal forward line.

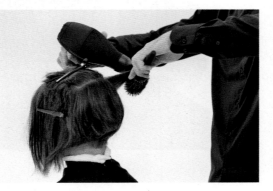

26 Continue this process into the sides and up to the side part. Lift the hair out from the base area according to the amount of base lift desired. Turn the ends and dry to bevel the ends slightly under.

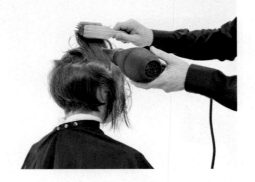

27 Finish blowdrying the front area, paying particular attention to the base area and mid-shaft. To create a smooth effect, grasp the ends in the brush and turn the ends downward.

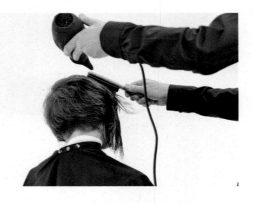

28 Once the hair is dry, detail the perimeter by starting at the nape and using the tips of the shears to point cut the edges of the perimeter to create softness. For a stronger line, blunt cut with the edges of your shears.

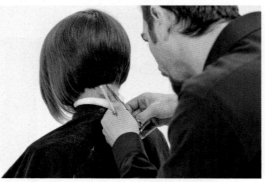

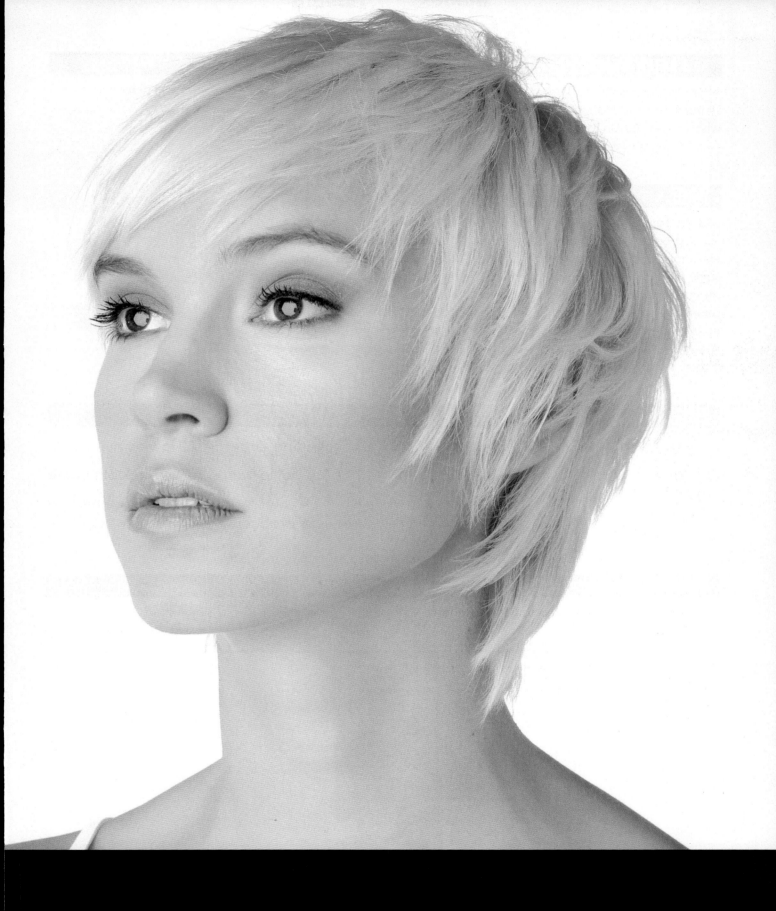

UNIFORM LAYERED HAIRCUT

LEARNING OBJECTIVES

After completing this section, you will be able to **perform** and **diagram** the Uniform Layered Haircut. You will also **understand** and be able to **identify** what makes the Uniform Layered Haircut uniform, how head shape directly controls the end result, and how the haircut is adjusted accordingly.

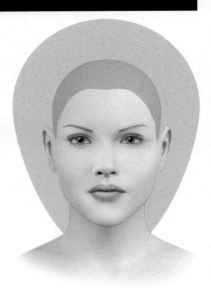

DESCRIPTION

Like the Long-Layered Haircut, the Uniform Layered Haircut is cut using 90 degrees of elevation; however instead of using a combination of elevations and overdirections, it is all cut at the same elevation and the same length. Your guide for this haircut is an interior traveling guideline – an interior guideline is one taken inside the haircut rather than on the perimeter. The resulting shape will appear soft and rounded, with no built-up weight or corners. The perimeter of the hair will fall softly, as the vertical sections in the interior reduce weight, while layers are used to release further weight and lend the hair movement and volume.

MATERIALS AND SUPPLIES

- ☐ Blowdryer
- ☐ Classic styling brush
- ☐ Cutting cape
- ☐ Cutting comb
- ☐ Haircutting shears
- ☐ Neck strip
- ☐ Paddle Brush
- ☐ Sectioning clips
- ☐ Spray bottle with water
- ☐ Styling product
- ☐ Towels
- ☐ Wide-tooth comb
- ☐ Mannequin or model

STEPS TO HAIRCUT

1 Carry out the **Guest Preparation Procedure**.

2 Detangle the hair using a wide-tooth comb.

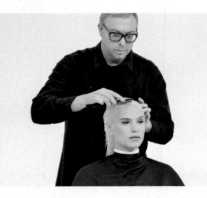

124

3 To create a guide, take a ½-inch (1.3-cm) wide, profile section from the front hairline to the nape. Cut using either a palm-to-palm or overhand cutting method. Make sure that your lines, sections, and partings are neat and balanced – use the mirror to ensure accuracy.

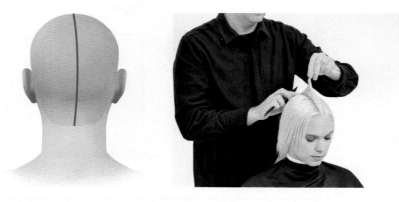

4 Starting at the nape, elevate the hair to 90 degrees and cut to the desired length, working in small increments following the head shape. It is very important that no overdirection is used during the entirety of the haircut, as any overdirecting will result in an inconsistent length.

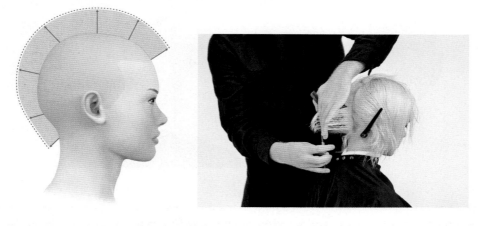

5 As you move up the section, cut to the second knuckle to avoid corners forming on the line. Follow the guide to the front hairline. Once you have cut the center guide, check the length for balance and remove any corners.

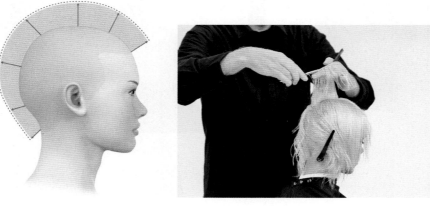

6. After completing the guide, take a horseshoe section from recession to recession and below the crown. Make sure your section is clean and balanced at both sides of the recession.

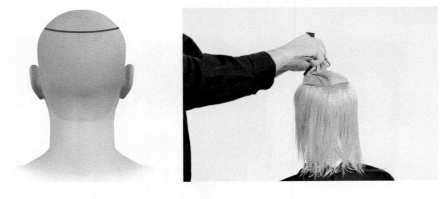

7. Take a horizontal parting from the occipital to the back of each ear and clip the section above your horizontal line. At the back, take a center section from the occipital to the nape, dividing your first profile section guide in half.

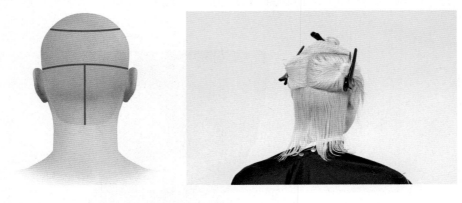

8. Starting at the center back, take a slightly diagonal forward parting through to the nape, incorporating your guide from the profile section.

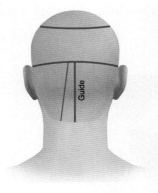
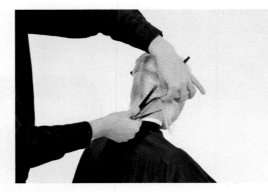

9 Elevate the hair to 90 degrees and cut parallel to the parting for your subsection, following the guide.

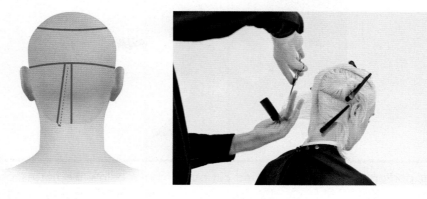

10 Cross-check horizontally on every fourth section. The line should be round because you are following the head shape.

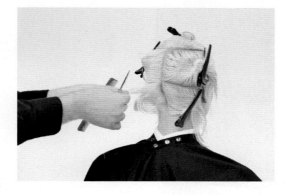

11 Continue taking slightly diagonal forward subsections, elevating at 90 degrees, and cutting parallel to your parting for your subsection until you have reached the back of the ear. Cross-check to show the uniform layer. Switch hand position and repeat on the opposite side.

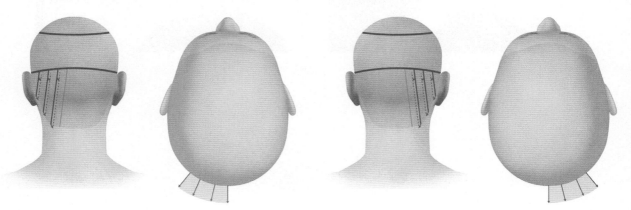

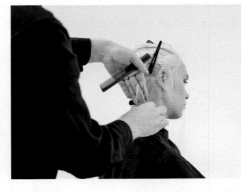

12 Release the lower portion of the horseshoe and cut palm-to-palm below the horseshoe on both sides. Continue taking slightly diagonal forward subsections, elevating at 90 degrees, and cutting parallel to your parting. Follow your guide until you have completed the side and then repeat on the opposite side. Cross-check back to front, checking the hair at the same elevation it was cut at.

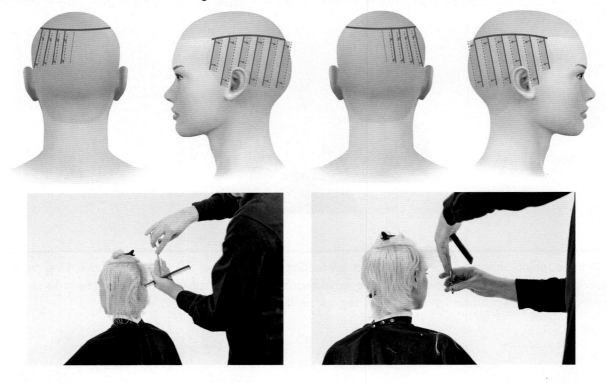

13 Release the remainder of the horseshoe section. Then take a radial section from above the crown to the top of each ear, separating the hair from front to back. Switch hand position and cut above your fingers for the remainder of the haircut.

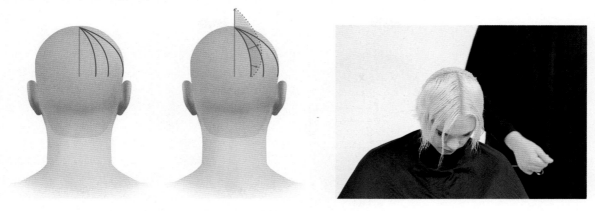

14 Pivoting (pie-shaped) sections are taken from below your radial section. Following your guide, elevate the hair at 90 degrees and cut until you have completed both sides.

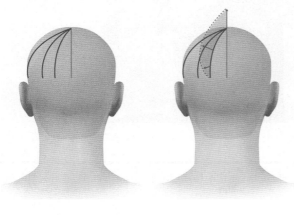

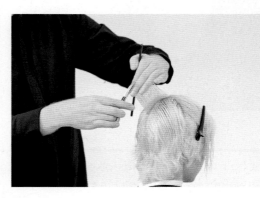

15 At this point, you should have a guide from the top, sides, and behind the radial section, allowing you to stay consistent and follow the head shape.

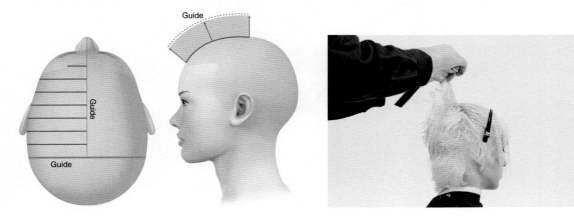

16 Continue by taking horizontal subsections, elevating at 90 degrees, and cutting with the traveling guide until you have reached the front hairline. Repeat the same technique on the opposite side, working your way from the bottom to the top of the head.

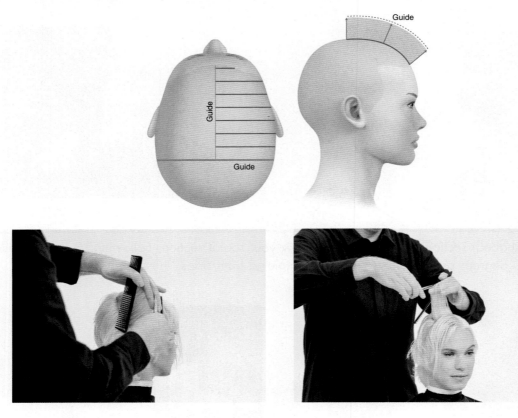

17 Dry the hair with your hands or a classic styling brush. Once the haircut is dry, texturize the interior to remove weight by using notching.

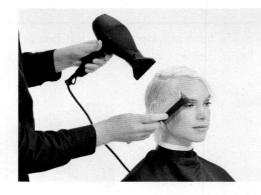

18 Hold the section 2 inches (5.1 cm) from the ends and enter the section parallel so you do not remove any length, working in 1-inch (2.5-cm) panels.

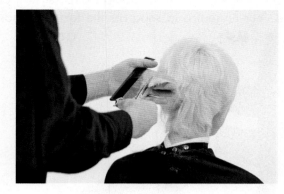

19 Use your mirror and look at the balance. Perform a fringe consultation and cut the bangs as desired. Detail the perimeter with point cutting and carving.

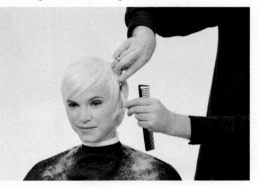

FINISH DESCRIPTION

The finished style is light and airy with soft, fringe-like lengths around the face. The key here is the minimal manipulation of the hair. If you blowdry the hair while moving it into place with your fingers, you will create a style that truly highlights the detailed texture within the haircut.

FINISH PREPARATION

Products play a key role when building versatility into a haircut, and a number of styling aids can be used to complete the finished look, depending upon the guest's hair and preference. A guest with fine-to-medium textured hair will benefit from the use of a thermal protectant and volumizing mousse layered together. Alternatively, thicker textures require more weight in the product, like a gel or a smoothing cream. A wax, serum, light oil, or aerosol hairspray can be used to complete the look and add definition, shine, and fullness.

20 Apply styling product and work it through the hair. Use a classic styling brush and blowdryer to gently move the hair into place. Use your fingertips to separate the textured ends.

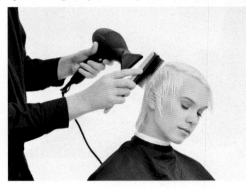

21 Use a small, rubber-based paddle brush to add fullness.

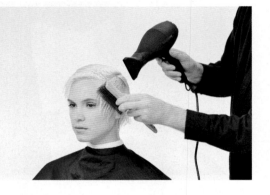

22 Use a use a classic styling or paddle brush around the face to add length and direction. The brush will add polish to the lengths. Alternate the brush with the fingers to accentuate texture.

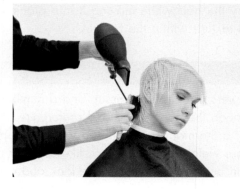

23 Use your fingertips to soften and personalize the design.

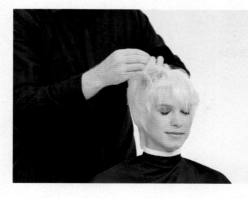

24 Finish with hairspray or a pomade for hold, separation, and texture.

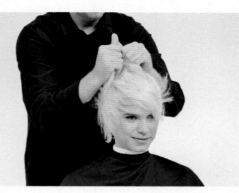

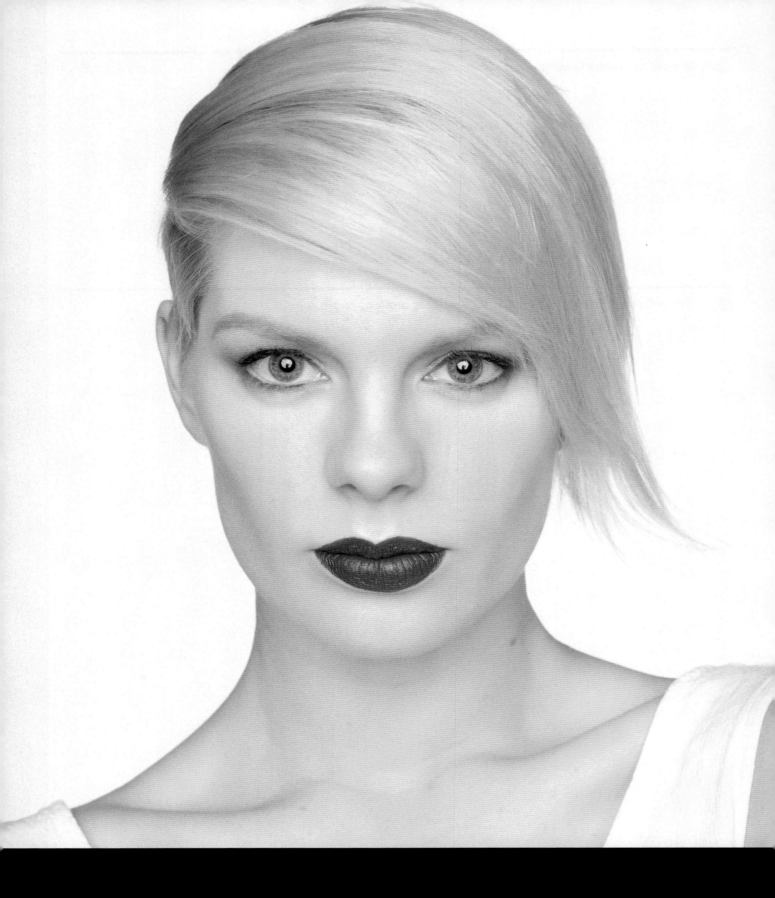

GRADUATED UNDERCUT

LEARNING OBJECTIVES

After completing this section, you will be able to **perform** and **diagram** the Graduated Undercut. You will also **understand** and be able to **identify** the Graduated Undercut by what makes a graduation heavy or light, as well as the difference between a graduation and a layer.

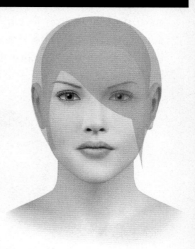

DESCRIPTION

The Graduated Undercut is a contemporary look achieved by combining aspects of two separate cuts. The underneath is cut utilizing short vertical graduation, first introduced in the Graduated Haircut, while the top is layered and left completely disconnected, as with the Disconnected Layers Haircut. The top horseshoe section must be placed above the round of the head; however, sectioning may need to be varied due to the size and density of guest hair in order to achieve proper balance. The haircut is then further customized to suit the guest's texture and individual lifestyle.

MATERIALS AND SUPPLIES

- ☐ Blowdryer
- ☐ Classic styling brush
- ☐ Cutting cape
- ☐ Cutting comb
- ☐ Flat iron
- ☐ Haircutting shears
- ☐ Neck strip
- ☐ Sectioning clips
- ☐ Spray bottle with water
- ☐ Styling product
- ☐ Towels
- ☐ Wide-tooth comb
- ☐ Mannequin or model

STEPS TO HAIRCUT

1 Carry out the **Guest Preparation Procedure**.

2 Detangle the hair using a wide-tooth comb.

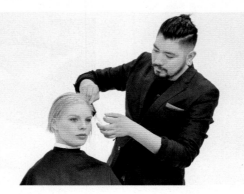

③ Place a horseshoe section from just above the occipital bone to the parietal ridge on both sides, as well as a profile section through the horseshoe to the nape. Isolate the hair above the horseshoe into two separate clips. At the sides, place a slightly diagonal back parting from the bottom of the horseshoe to behind each ear. Secure the hair behind the ear in back into two clips. Make sure that your sectioning is neat and balanced — use the mirror to ensure accuracy.

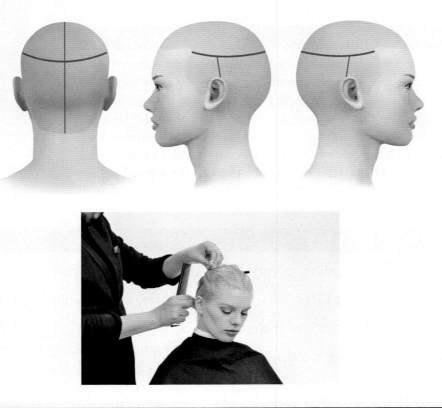

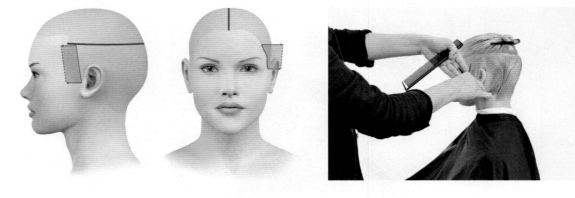

④ Begin at the side by creating a ½-inch (1.3-cm) wide, diagonal back subsection from the parietal ridge to the side burn. Elevate the hair out at 90 degrees and cut your line approximately 1 to 1½ inches (2.5 to 3.8 cm) in length, with your fingers parallel to your part. This length will vary depending on suitability and the lifestyle of the guest.

5 Take another ½-inch (1.3-cm) wide, slightly diagonal back subsection, elevate the hair at 90 degrees, and cut the line following your guide from the previously cut section. As you work, comb away the previously cut sections, maintaining your guide and cross-checking every third subsection to ensure balance in your line.

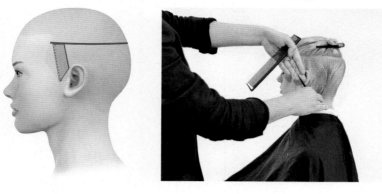

6 Repeat this technique until you have reached the parting behind the ear. Once there, switch body position and repeat the same technique on the opposite side of the head, stopping in the same place. Check for balance and make any adjustments necessary before moving on.

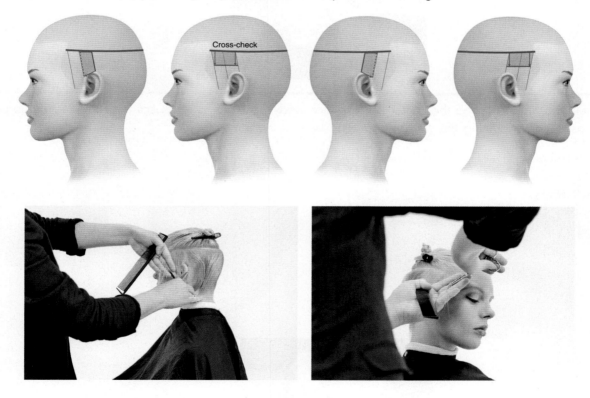

7 When the cross-check is complete, switch body positions, and move back to the side where you started. Here you will release the hair behind the ear and continue cutting until you reach the center back. To ensure consistency in your cutting line and elevation, subdivide your subsections as you work, following and traveling with your guide from the previously cut section.

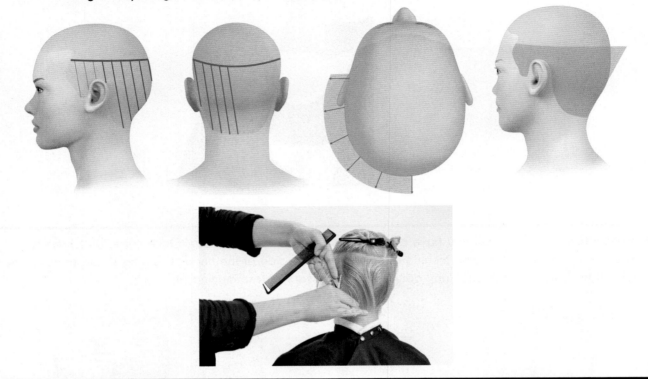

8 When you have reached the center back, switch body positions, and repeat the same technique on the opposite side, resuming the cut at the parting behind the ear.

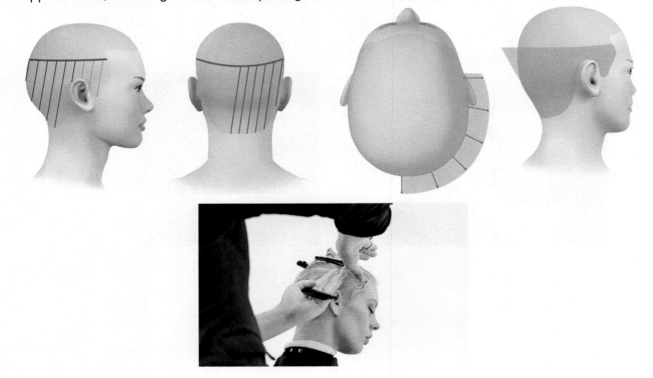

9 Once you reach the center back on the opposite side, overlap your slightly diagonal partings to ensure that you have blended your graduation with the other side.

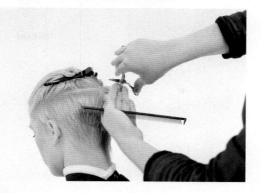

10 Take a moment to soften your lines on both sides and remove weight by utilizing notching. Carving can also be used to give separation and direction to the hair.

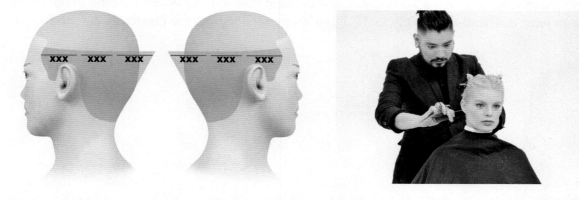

11 Use the mirror and turn the chair around, looking for balance, texture, and proper weight removal. Release the horseshoe section and remoisten the top section if necessary. At the back, elevate the hair and soften the graduation line and perimeter with notching.

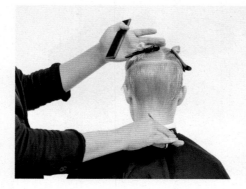

12 Create an arc section, by taking a curved parting from the top of each ear across the crown and a straight parting from the top of each ear through the occipital. Secure all hair below the arc section out of the way with clips, as the bottom is disconnected from the graduation.

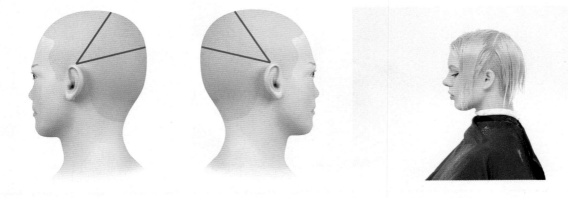

13 At the top of the arc, take a ½-inch (1.3-cm) wide, pivoting or pie-shaped subsection extending to the occipital. Elevate the hair out at 90 degrees and cut your layers with the round of the head. Make sure to leave at least a 4- to 5-inch (10.2- to 12.7-cm) disconnection from the previously cut graduation.

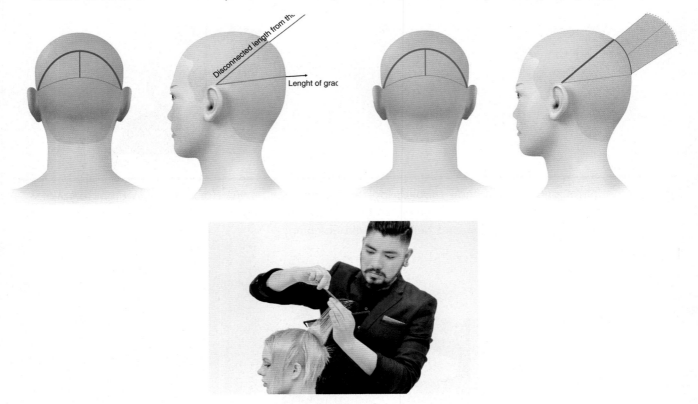

14 Take another ½-inch (1.3-cm) wide, pivoting or pie-shaped subsection, elevate the hair straight out at 90 degrees and cut your layers with the round of the head, following your guide from the previously cut section. Continue this technique until you have reached above the ear.

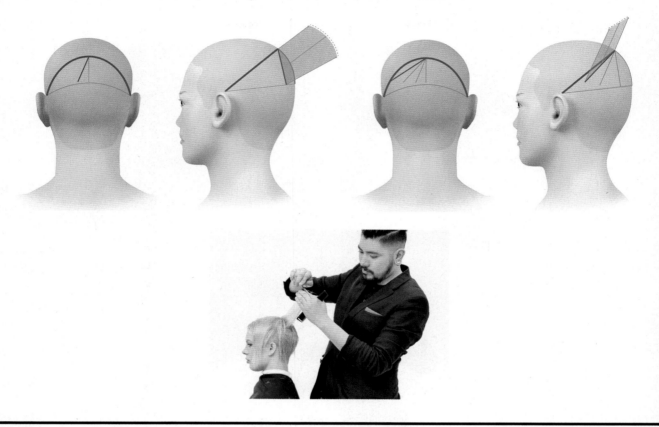

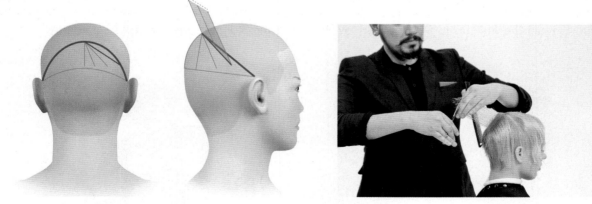

15 Switch body position and repeat Steps 13 to 14 on the opposite side.

16 The hair at the top will be cut in an asymmetric manner, giving a light and a heavy side to the part over the eye. At the top, create a stationary guide by placing a ½-inch (1.3-cm) wide, pivoting section diagonally from the crown to the corner of one eye. Using the length of your crown as a guide, elevate the hair straight up to 90 degrees and cut your layers square – approximately 5 to 6 inches (12.7 to 15.2 cm) in length – from the crown to the corner of the eye.

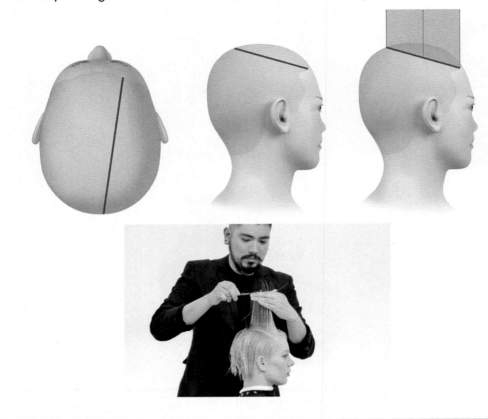

17 Working the side opposite of your body, place another ½-inch (1.3-cm) wide, pivoting or pie-shaped section. Elevate the hair up to 90 degrees, overdirect to the stationary guide, and cut square.

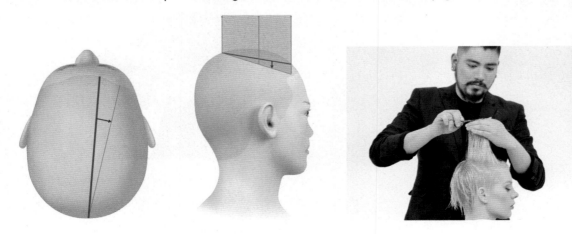

18 Continue taking ½-inch (1.3-cm) wide, pivoting sections, elevating the hair up to 90 degrees, overdirecting to the stationary guide and cutting square. Repeat until you have cut all the remaining hair in that section.

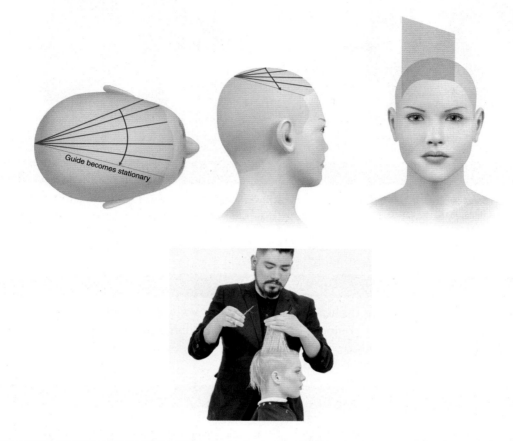

19 Moving to the other side of the guest, place another ½-inch (1.3-cm) wide, pivoting subsection from the crown to the light side of the stationary guide. Elevate the hair up to 90 degrees, overdirect to the stationary guide, and cut square. Repeat this technique until the side is complete. You will notice the top layers are slightly asymmetric – this was achieved by overdirecting the hair to the stationary guide, from the crown to the corner of the eye.

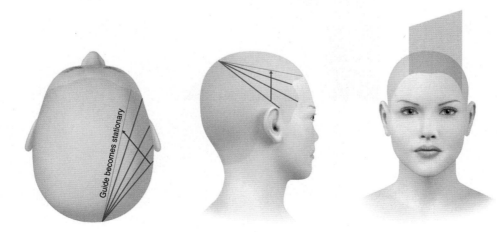

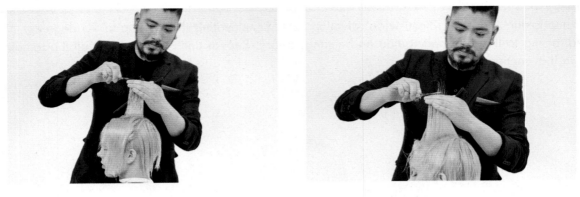

FINISH DESCRIPTION

This shape should expose shorter graduation underneath a longer, slightly asymmetric top section. The haircut should visually look blended but technically disconnected. This style works best on straight to wavy hair.

FINISH PREPARATION

To bring the most out of this shape, use a classic styling brush for volume and then flat iron for smoothness and texture, finishing with a texturizing pomade. Work the product through the hair, exposing the shorter undercut by tucking the hair behind the ear.

STEPS TO FINISH

20 Apply a volumizing mousse and a thermal protectant, combing through for even distribution. Blowdry the hair with a classic styling brush.

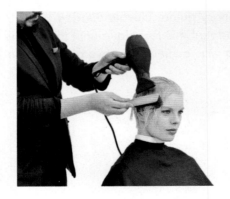

21 Once completely dry, take ½-inch (1.3-cm) panels and flat iron the hair straight. The top should be worn to the heavier side with a **Side Swept Bang (Fringe)**.

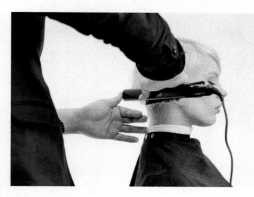

22 If further texturizing is needed, you can use notching, carving, or slicing, working in 1-inch (2.5-cm) panels on the top. Detail the perimeter with scissor-over-comb or point cutting. Finish by applying a texturizing pomade to give shape, shine, volume, separation, and texture.

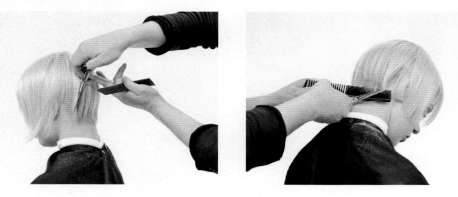

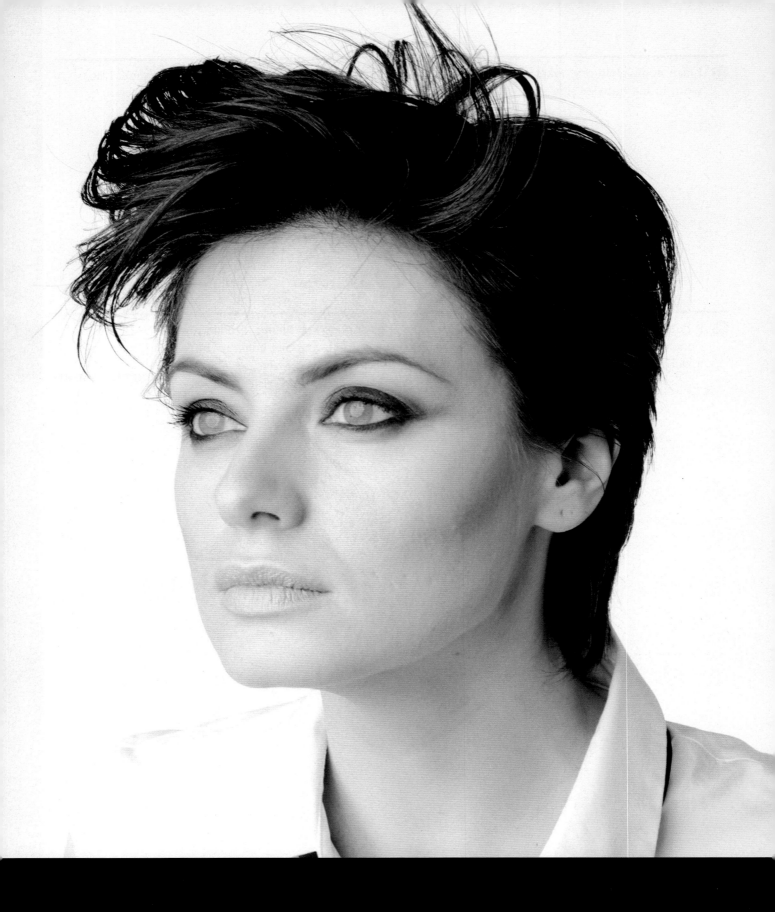

DISCONNECTED LAYERS

5 Take a ½-inch (1.3-cm) wide, pivoting subsection from the crown to the nape. Elevate the hair straight out at 90 degrees and cut, following the guide from the previously cut section.

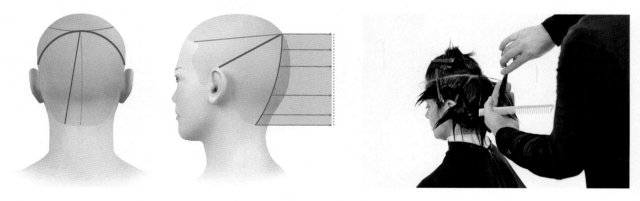

6 Continue taking ½-inch (1.3-cm) wide, pivoting subsections from the crown to the nape, elevating the hair straight out at 90 degrees, and cutting your layers. Follow your traveling guide from the previously cut section.

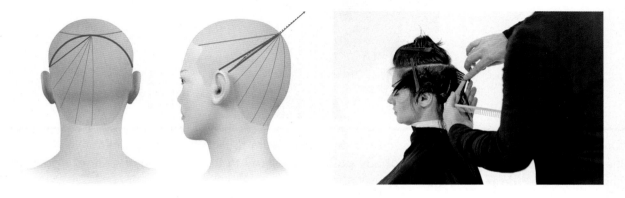

7 When you reach the parting at the top of the ear, cross-check and then repeat the same technique on the opposite side of your profile parting. Before moving on, check for balance in the back between the two sides.

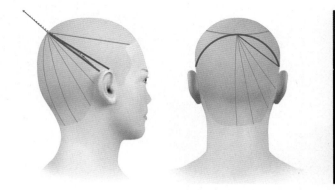
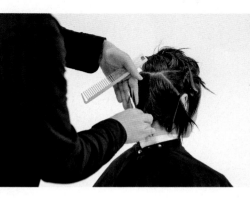

8 Once you reach the side section at the top of the other ear section, change from pivoting to traveling diagonal forward subsections, to help maintain length at the bottom of the hairline. Continue to take ½-inch (1.3-cm) wide subsections, elevate the hair straight out at 90 degrees, and cut until you reach the front hairline.

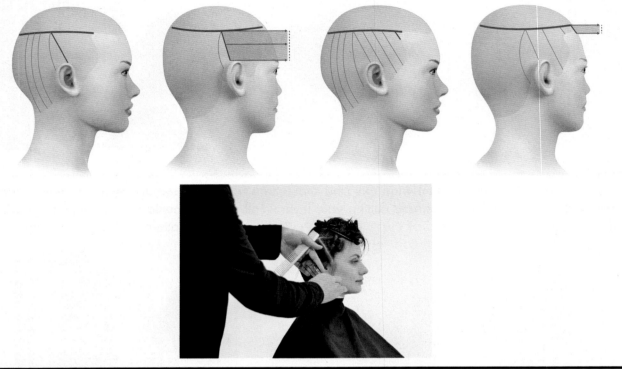

9 Once you have completed one side, cross-check, then return to the first section and continue working the opposite side the same way. Our body position continues to be behind each section. Again, cross-check once the side is complete.

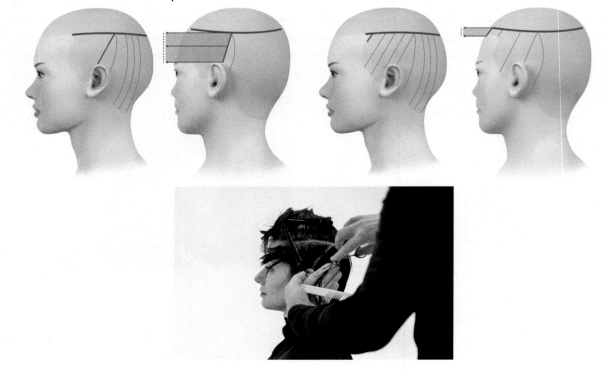

10. Once you have completed the layers underneath the horseshoe, blowdry the hair straight and smooth with a classic styling brush, working in ½-inch (1.3-cm) subsections.

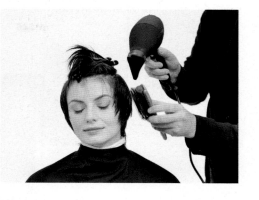

11. When the hair has been completely dried, clean up the hairline if needed and begin to remove weight by utilizing notching and/or carving. Elevate the hair with the comb and soften your interior and perimeter with notching. Combine this with the carving technique – or alternatively, slide cutting – throughout the sides to give the hair separation and movement.

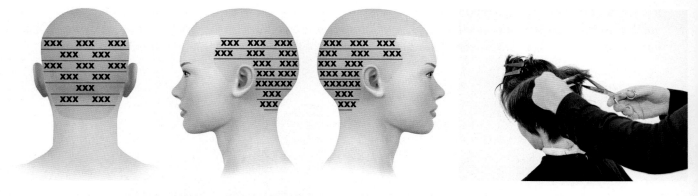

12. Release the top section and remoisten the top if necessary. Place a ½-inch (1.3-cm) wide, profile section from the front hairline to the crown. Taking your guide from the crown, elevate the hair straight up to 90 degrees and cut your layers from short to long – approximately 4 inches (10.2 cm) at the crown to 5 to 6 inches (12.7 to 15.2 cm) at the front hairline.

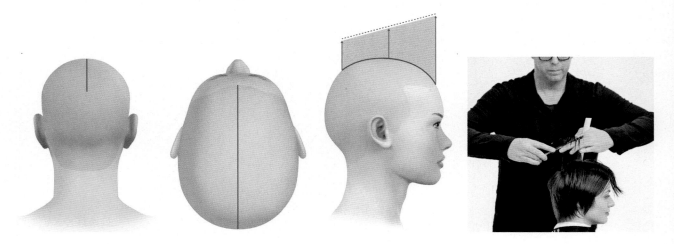

13 Take a ½-inch (1.3-cm) wide, pivoting section from the crown through the front hairline. Elevate your section up to 90 degrees and overdirect to the center, following your guide from the previously cut section and cutting from the crown through the front hairline.

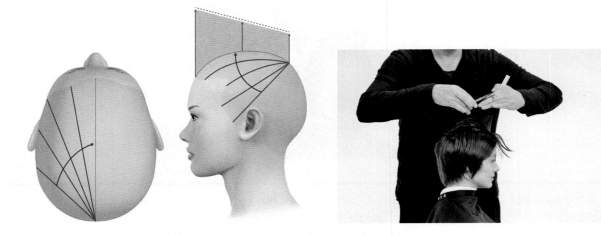

14 Continue this approach until you have completed one side. When cutting the other side, you will remain in the same body and hand positions. When cutting from this position, your guide (taken from the first section) will be on the opposite side of the section. Work from the crown through the front as you did before. Once this section is complete, cross-check to ensure the interior of the cut is shorter than the exterior.

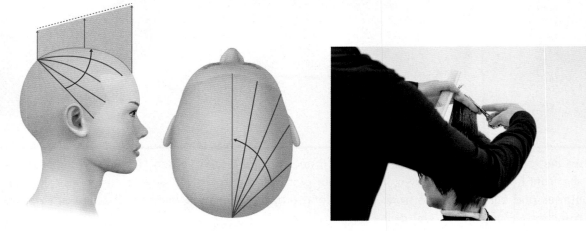

15 If more texture in the hair is desired after completing the cut, texturize the hair by taking one inch horizontal sections throughout the top and point cutting the hair to remove weight and add texture. Texturize around the perimeter with point cutting.

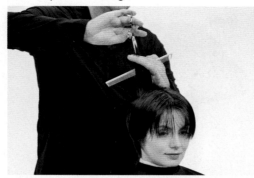

16 Perform a fringe consultation and cut the bangs as desired.

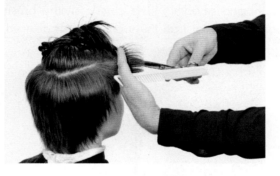

FINISH DESCRIPTION

This shape should have a visual disconnection between the short, round layers and the longer, disconnected top. It can be worn back off the face in a pompadour or with a side-swept fringe, allowing your guest to dress it up for the occasion.

FINISH PREPARATION

Your products will change depending on the finish. For a smoother look, use a thermal protectant and smoothing cream, then finish with a serum. For an edgier look, use a gel for a pompadour finish, or blowdry and finish with wax or texturizing pomade to expose all of the cut's texture.

17 Apply a small amount of smoothing cream and a thermal protectant to the hair, comb through for even distribution.

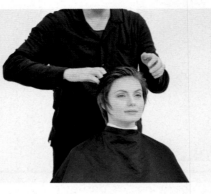

18 Blowdry the top section straight and smooth with a classic styling brush. Once the hair is completely dry, take ½-inch (1.3-cm) panels and flat iron the top section if desired.

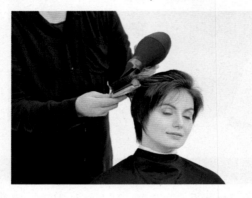

19 Finish by applying a wax or texturing pomade – this will expose the texture and add separation and movement.

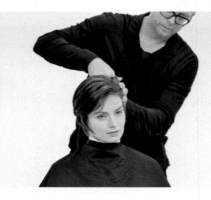

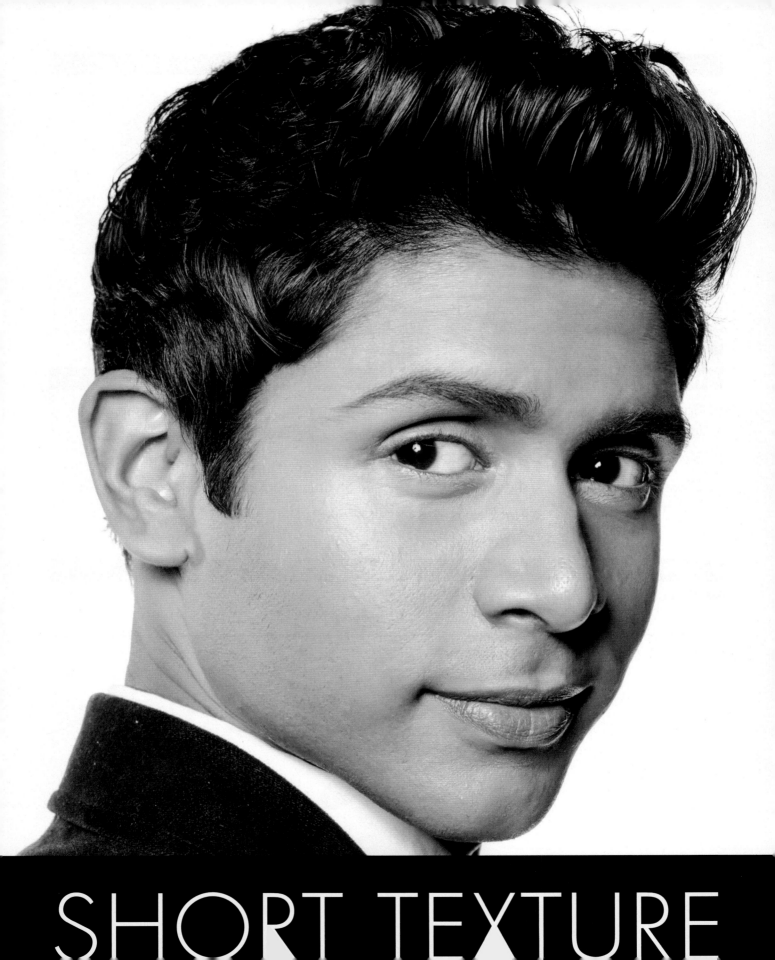

SHORT TEXTURE

After completing this section, you will be able to **perform** and **diagram** the Short Texture haircut. You will also **understand** and be able to **identify** whom the Short Texture haircut would benefit the most and why, as well as the difference between final looks created with scissors and those with clippers.

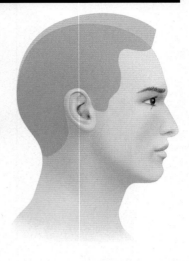

DESCRIPTION

This classic masculine shape is modernized by combining scissor-over-comb and advanced texturizing techniques. Like the Disconnected Layers haircut, Short Texture uses scissor-over-comb and round layers in the crown, cut at a 90-degree elevation, to create a more lived-in look. This is in stark contrast to clipper-over-comb or clipper work in general, which creates a more aggressive, clean-cut look. The end result here is a versatile, low maintenance, cropped haircut suitable for men of all ages. Taper is optional.

MATERIALS AND SUPPLIES

- ☐ Barbering comb (optional)
- ☐ Blowdryer
- ☐ Classic styling brush
- ☐ Cutting cape
- ☐ Cutting comb
- ☐ Haircutting shears
- ☐ Neck strip
- ☐ Sectioning clips
- ☐ Spray bottle with water
- ☐ Styling product
- ☐ Towels
- ☐ Trimmers
- ☐ Wide-tooth comb
- ☐ Mannequin or model

STEPS TO HAIRCUT

1 Carry out the **Guest Preparation Procedure**.

2 Detangle the hair using a wide-tooth comb.

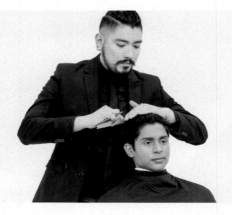

3 Begin by placing a horseshoe section from just below the crown to the parietal ridge on both sides. Isolate the hair at the top with sectioning clips. Make sure that your lines, sections, and partings are neat and balanced – use the mirror to ensure accuracy.

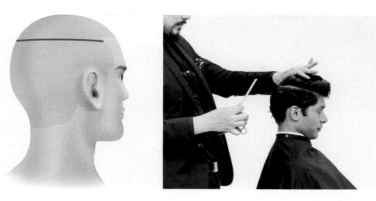

4 Take a 2-inch (5.1-cm) subsection, in both width and length, below the horseshoe at the crown. Comb the hair from underneath, holding the section lengthwise, and elevate at 90 degrees from the head and parallel to the horseshoe section. Cut the hair to approximately 2 inches (5.1 cm) in length.

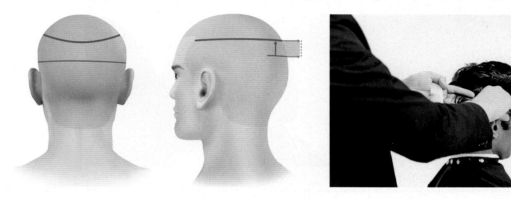

5 Take another 2-inch (5.1-cm) subsection from below the horseshoe at the crown. Repeat the cutting technique by combing the hair from underneath, holding the section lengthwise, and elevating at 90 degrees from the head and parallel to the horseshoe section.

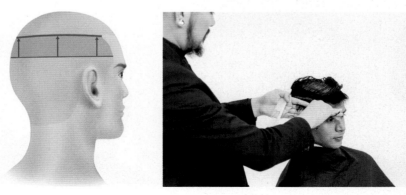

6 Continue this technique until you reach the front hairline. Switch body positions and repeat on the opposite side, starting adjacent to your first subsection at the crown. Make sure that your 2-inch (5.1-cm) subsections, elevation, and line are consistent and balanced as you move around the head.

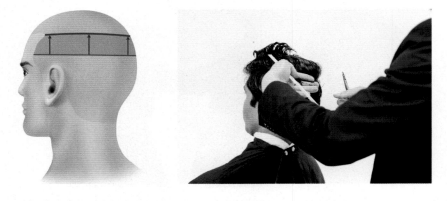

7 There should be no corners on your 2-inch (5.1-cm) subsection – it should mimic the horseshoe section. This subsection will serve as your guide for the entire haircut.

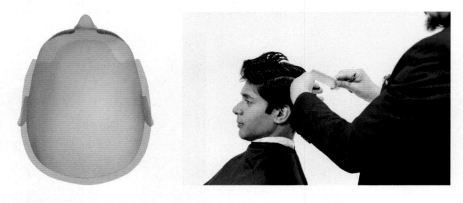

8 Once you have completed cutting your 2-inch (5.1-cm) subsection, place a ½-inch (1.3-cm) wide, vertical section from the crown to the nape, elevate the hair straight out from the head at 90 degrees, and cut your line. For control and easier handling, you will subdivide the subsection, holding in your hand only as much hair as you are able to cut.

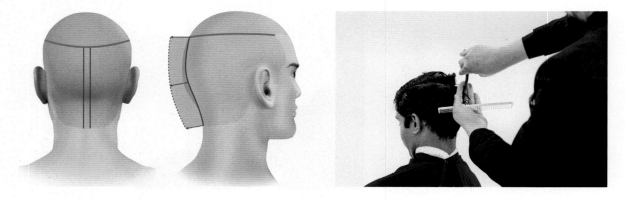

9 Continue by taking ½-inch (1.3-cm) wide, vertical subsections, elevating the hair straight out from the head at 90 degrees and cutting, following your guide from the previously cut section. Repeat this technique until you have completed one side.

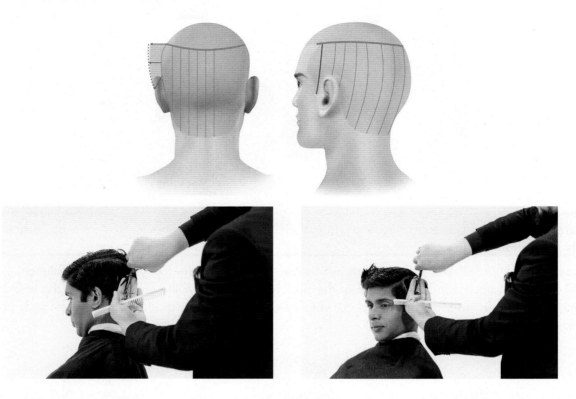

10 Switch body position and repeat on the opposite side of the head.

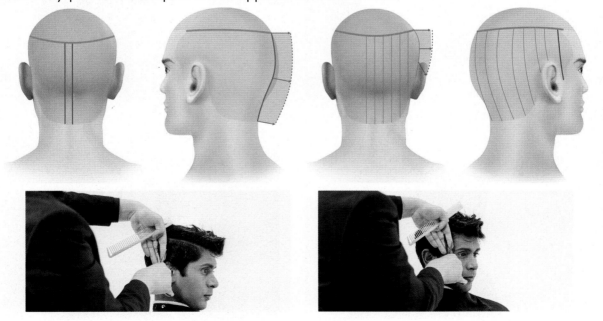

11 Once you have completed layering the hair below the horseshoe, release the top section and create a band section from the center of the forehead to just below the crown. Elevate the hair up to 90 degrees from the head and cut a layer with the round of the head, following your guide from the previously cut section below the crown.

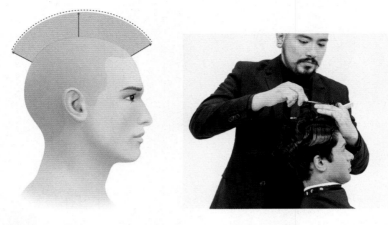

12 Place a diagonal forward parting from just below the crown to the top of each ear. Take a ½-inch (1.3-cm) wide subsection from the top of the parting to just below the crown. Elevate the hair straight out at 90 degrees from the head and cut your line, following your guide from the previously cut section below the crown.

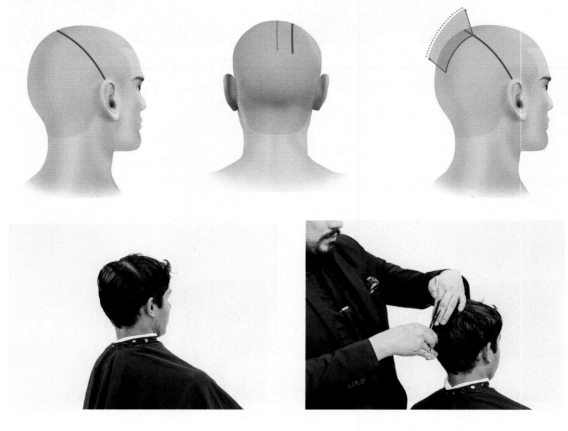

13 Continue this approach until you reach the parting at the top of the ear. Switch body position and repeat the same technique on the opposite side.

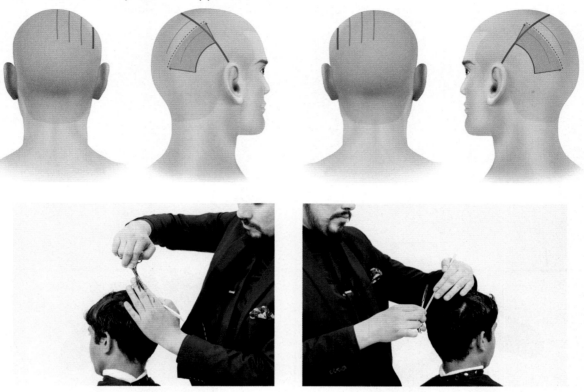

14 To complete the top, start at the crown and create a horizontal subsection extending past the parietal ridge. Elevate the hair straight up to 90 degrees and cut square, following the guide from the previously cut section at the center and behind the parting at the top of the ear.

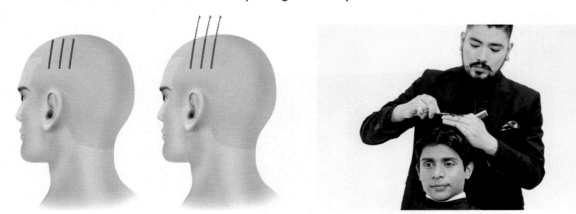

15 Continue taking horizontal subsections from the top, extending them past the parietal ridge, elevating the hair up at 90 degrees, and cutting your line. Follow your traveling guide from the previously cut section. Carry this technique through the top and parietal ridge of both sides.

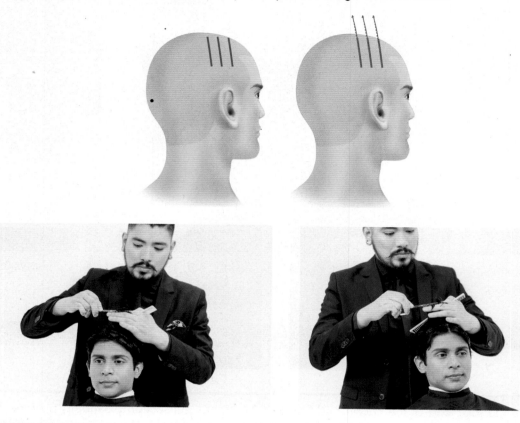

16 With a taper, scissor-over-comb your perimeter. Starting at the back, begin at the nape, place your comb at the hairline, and scissor-over-comb up approximately 2 inches (5.1 cm), increasing in length as you move up from the hairline. Repeat the same technique at the sides and perimeter. Then clean up the hairline and sideburns with trimmers.

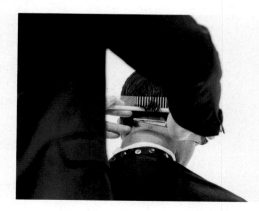

17. Without a taper, strengthen your line with scissors, then clean up the perimeter by using trimmers. If needed, texturize the interior and remove weight by using carving, notching, and slicing.

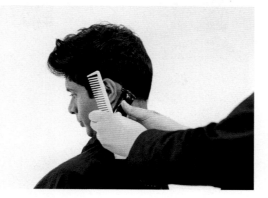

FINISH DESCRIPTION

This short, masculine shape has options when it comes to styling, and the textured interior allows for versatility and movement.

FINISH PREPARATION

When it comes to styling, men typically want low-maintenance haircuts. Products of choice for this look are a gel (for a wet look or tuxedo side part), wax (for a matte finish and texture), and texturizing pomade (for an edgier, disheveled look).

STEPS TO FINISH

18. Apply a medium-hold gel to the hair and blowdry straight with a classic styling brush. Once the hair is completely dry you can begin to detail and texturize the shape.

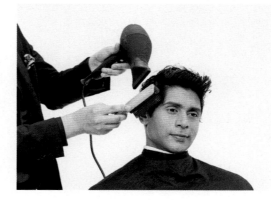

19 Enhance the shape by applying a light hold wax for a matte finish and to expose the texture.

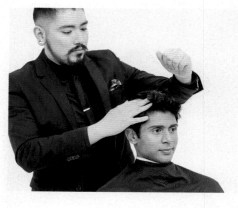

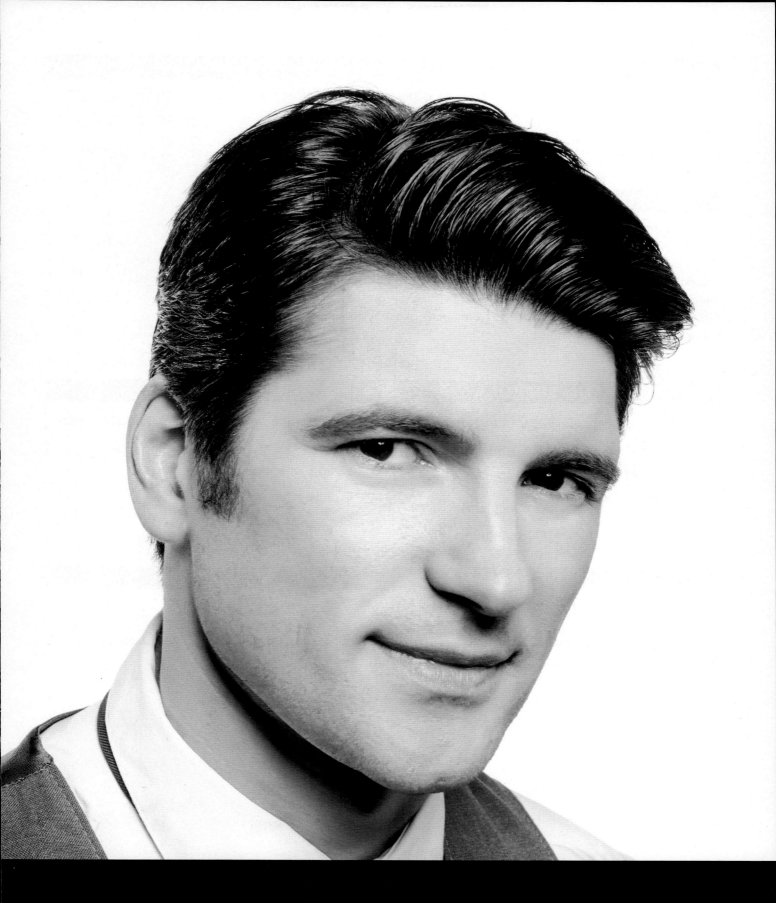

SQUARE LAYERS

LEARNING OBJECTIVES

After completing this section, you will be able to **perform** and **diagram** the Square Layers haircut. You will also **understand** and be able to **identify** what makes the layers of Square Layers square, and how Square Layers creates a result that will flatter any guest's head shape.

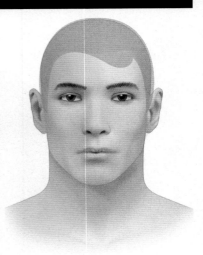

DESCRIPTION

Thanks to how the hair is texturized, Square Layers can easily be transformed from business to casual, creating options for the contemporary male. Like the Graduated Undercut, this haircut uses diagonal back subsections on the sides and back with a 90 degree elevation. In addition, the crown is cut with the round of the head, using an arc section. Where the two differ is in how Square Layers enhances guest head shape, stays short, and lacks a disconnection.

MATERIALS AND SUPPLIES

- ☐ Barbering comb (optional)
- ☐ Blow dryer
- ☐ Classic styling brush
- ☐ Cutting cape
- ☐ Cutting comb
- ☐ Haircutting shears
- ☐ Neck strip
- ☐ Sectioning clips
- ☐ Spray bottle with water
- ☐ Styling product
- ☐ Towels
- ☐ Trimmers
- ☐ Wide-tooth comb
- ☐ Mannequin or model

STEPS TO HAIRCUT

1 Carry out the **Guest Preparation Procedure**.

2 Detangle the hair using a wide-tooth comb.

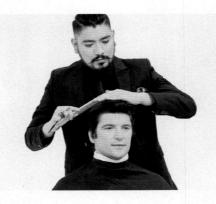

3 Begin by placing a horseshoe section from just below the crown to the recession area on both sides. Isolate the hair at the top with sectioning clips. At the sides, place a slightly diagonal back parting from the bottom of the horseshoe to behind each ear. Make sure that your lines, sections, and partings are neat and balanced — use the mirror to ensure accuracy.

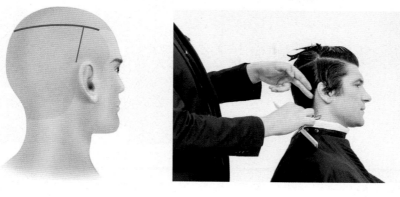

4 Starting at a side, take a ½-inch (1.3-cm) wide, slightly diagonal back subsection in the front hairline extending from the parietal ridge through the sideburn, in front of the ear. Elevate the hair straight out at 90 degrees from the head and cut your line square, approximately 2 to 3 inches (5.1 to 7.6 cm) in length.

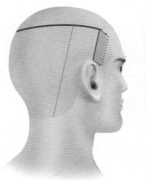
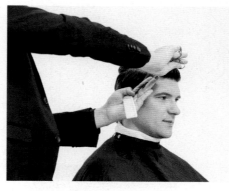

5 Take a ½-inch (1.3-cm) wide, slightly diagonal back subsection, elevate the hair straight out at 90 degrees and cut square, following a traveling guide from the previously cut section. Continue taking ½-inch (1.3-cm) wide, diagonal back subsections, elevating the hair straight out at 90 degrees and cutting your line square, traveling with your previously cut section as a guide. Repeat this technique until you have reached the parting behind the ear.

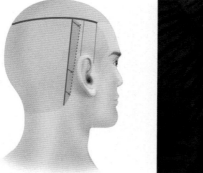
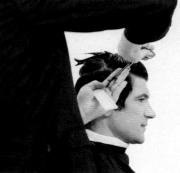

6 Switch body positions and repeat on the opposite side of the head, starting at the front hairline. Once you cut your first section, check your balance with the opposite side before continuing.

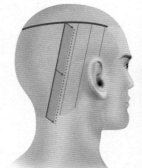
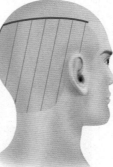
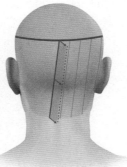

7 When the cross-check is complete, switch body positions and move back to the side where you started. Here you will release the hair behind the ear and continue cutting until you reach the center back. To ensure consistency in your cutting line and elevation, subdivide your subsections as you work, following and traveling with your guide from the previously cut section.

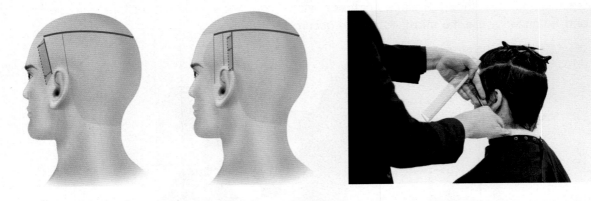

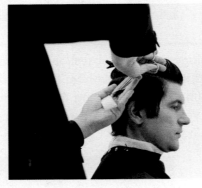

8 When you have reached the center back, switch body positions and repeat the same technique on the opposite side, resuming the cut at the parting behind the ear.

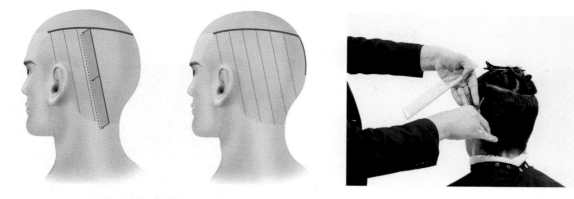

9 Once you reach the center back on the opposite side, overlap your slightly diagonal partings to ensure that you have blended one side with the other side.

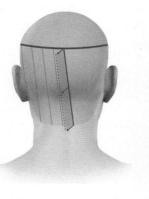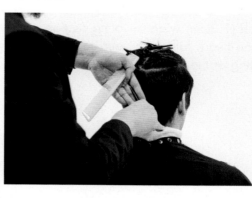

10 Release the top section, then create an arc section, by taking a curved parting from the top of each ear across the crown and a straight parting from the top of each ear through the occipital. Secure all hair below the arc section out of the way with clips.

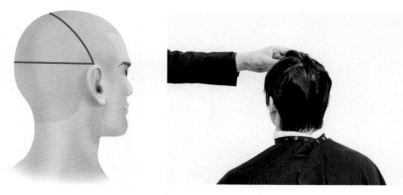

11 At the top of the arc, take a ½-inch (1.3-cm) wide, pivoting section extending to the occipital. Elevate the hair out at 90 degrees and cut your layers with the round of the head, following your guide from the previously cut section underneath.

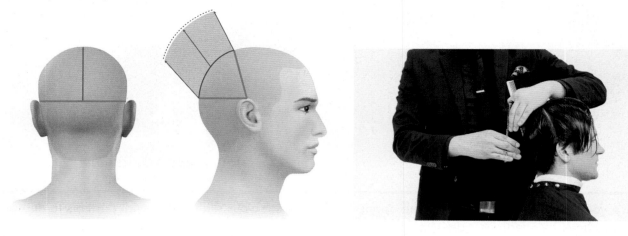

12 Take another ½-inch (1.3-cm) wide, pivoting section, elevate the hair straight out at 90 degrees, and cut with the round of the head, following your guide from the previously cut section. Continue this approach through to the parting at the ear.

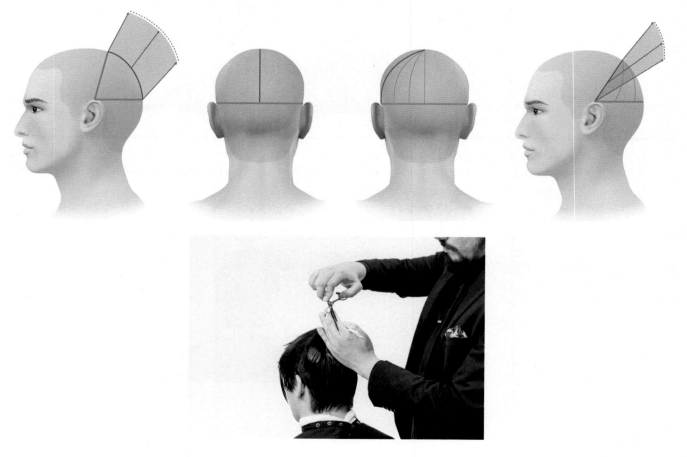

13 Switch body positions and repeat the same technique on the opposite side, starting in the center back.

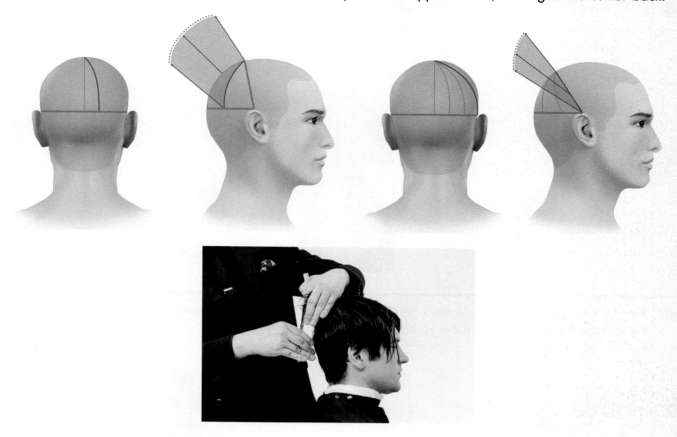

14 Once the layering in the crown is complete, the top of head will be divided by placing a parting from the center of the forehead to the crown and then from the crown to each ear.

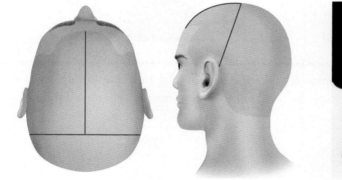

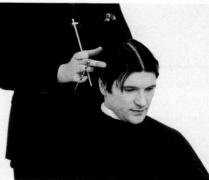

15 At the crown, take a ½-inch (1.3-cm) wide section from the center of the forehead to the crown and elevate the hair straight up at 90 degrees from the head then cut square, using your previously cut section at the crown as a guide to length.

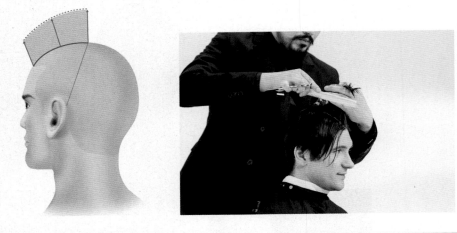

16 Next, on your dominant side, take a ½-inch (1.3-cm) wide, horizontal subsection. Elevate the hair straight up to 90 degrees and cut your line square, using your previously cut section from the crown and center as a guide.

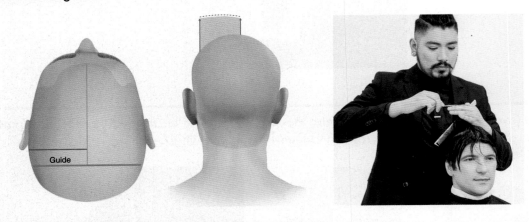

17 Continue to take ½-inch (1.3-cm) wide, horizontal subsections, elevate the hair straight up, and cut your line square, using you previously cut section as a traveling guide. Follow this technique until you reach the front hairline.

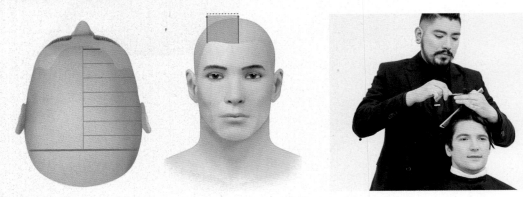

18 Repeat on the opposite side, starting in the crown.

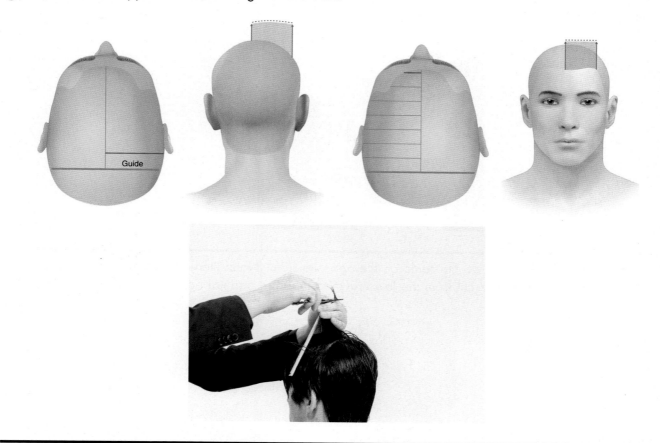

19 Once you have completed the top section, part the hair from the center of the forehead to the apex and place a radial section from the apex to each ear. Beginning at the front parietal ridge on your dominant front side, take a ½-inch (1.3-cm) wide, slightly diagonal back subsection, elevate the hair straight out at 90 degrees, and cut your square using your guide from the sides. (Note: Here you also have the option to stand behind the guest and cut from the low crown to the front parietal ridge.)

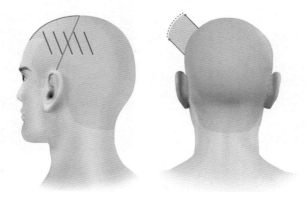

20 Repeat this technique from the parietal ridge at the front hairline until you reach the radial section at the top of the ear.

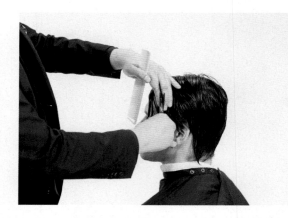

21 Switch body positions and do the same on the opposite side. (Note: Here you also have the option to stand behind the guest and cut from the low crown to the front parietal ridge.)

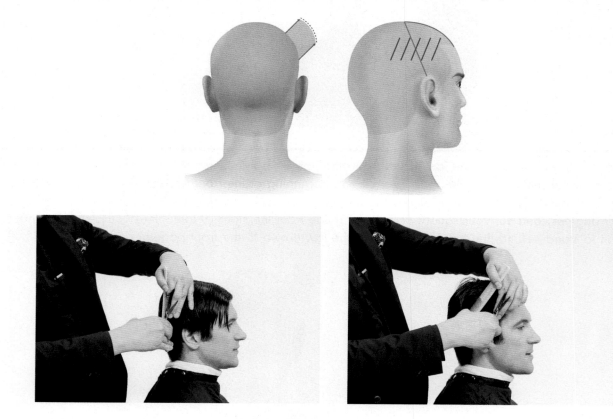

22 At the perimeter, you have two options: You can either point cut for a textured line, or blunt cut to add strength to the line. Depending on the length at the sides, the hair should either be above the ear or partially covering it.

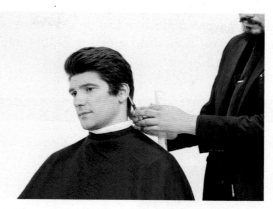

23 Once you complete the perimeter and the hair is totally dry, use your trimmer to clean up the neckline and sideburns. If needed, texturize the entire interior by taking 1-inch (2.5-cm) panels and notching. This will remove weight, soften your lines, and add movement and texture for versatility.

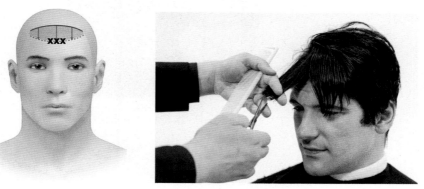

24 At the front, comb the bangs forward and point cut your line slightly round.

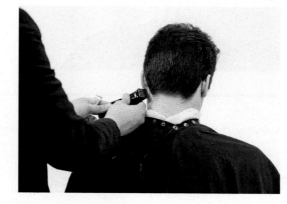

FINISH DESCRIPTION

This shape is ideal for the businessman who wants a conservative style by day and a fashion-forward look by night. The square layers enhance the head shape, while the texture in the interior provides versatility.

FINISH PREPARATION

Men's haircuts should be low maintenance when it comes to styling, and most prefer not to have to blowdry their hair. Use a classic styling brush for a styled look or your fingers for a lived-in look. Products of choice for this look are a gel (for a wet-looking pompadour or tuxedo side part), wax (for a matte finish and texture), texturizing pomade (for an edgier, disheveled look), or a light-hold pomade (for shine, movement, and separation).

STEPS TO FINISH

25 Apply a light mousse and a thermal protectant spray, comb through for even distribution.

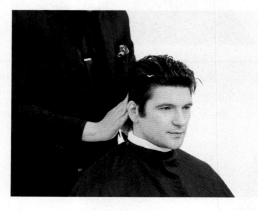

26 Blowdry the hair with a classic styling brush, fingers, or comb, depending on if a lived-in look is desired. Once the hair is completely dry, begin to detail and texturize the shape.

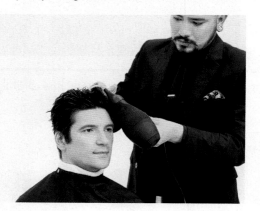

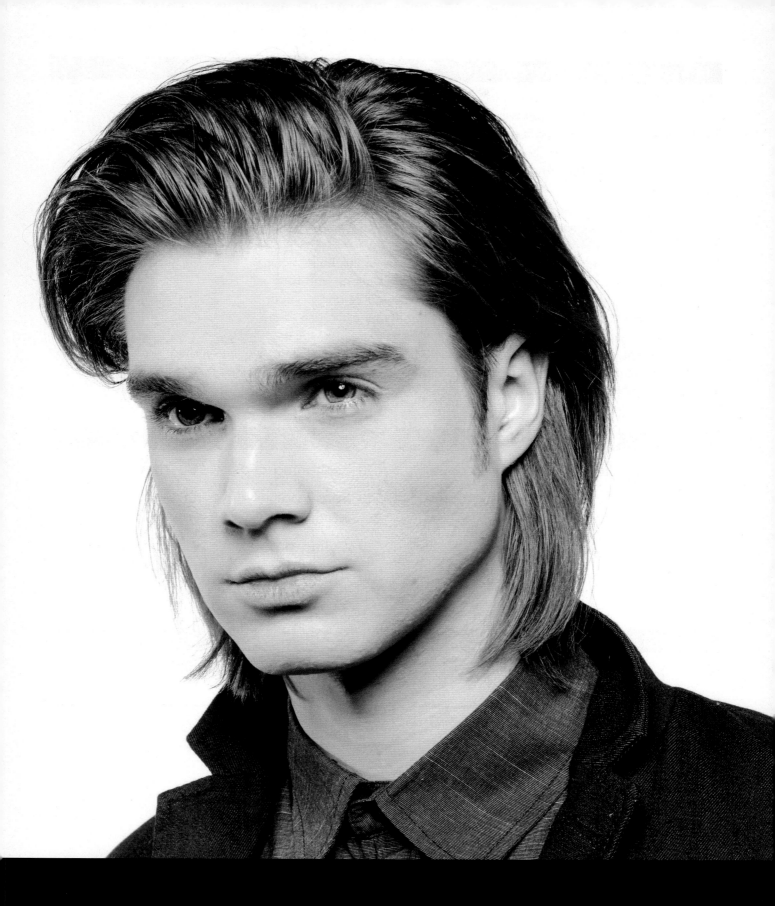

VERSATILE MOVEMENT

LEARNING OBJECTIVES

After completing this section, you will be able to **perform** and **diagram** the Versatile Movement haircut. You will also **understand** and be able to **identify** the differences among the Uniform, Long-Layered, and Versatile Movement haircuts, particularly how the use of elevation and layering affects the versatility of the end result, and how the haircut can be adjusted for a man or a woman.

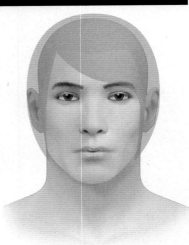

DESCRIPTION

Designed for mid-length and shorter hair, the versatility of this haircut comes from its approach to layering and texturizing. Like the Uniform and Long-Layered Haircuts, Versatile Movement uses a traveling guide and is cut at a 90-degree elevation. Versatile Movement takes a different approach to the layering process from there. The layering technique used with versatile movement creates an end result allowing for multiple ways to wear and style the finished look. The finished look is a modern shag, combining strength, and texture within the lines to create a style that is the perfect look for the fashion-forward male.

MATERIALS AND SUPPLIES

- ☐ Barbering comb (optional)
- ☐ Blowdryer
- ☐ Classic styling brush
- ☐ Cutting cape
- ☐ Cutting comb
- ☐ Haircutting shears
- ☐ Neck strip
- ☐ Sectioning clips
- ☐ Spray bottle with water
- ☐ Styling product
- ☐ Towels
- ☐ Trimmers
- ☐ Wide-tooth comb
- ☐ Mannequin or model

STEPS TO HAIRCUT

1 Carry out the **Guest Preparation Procedure**.

2 Detangle the hair using a wide-tooth comb.

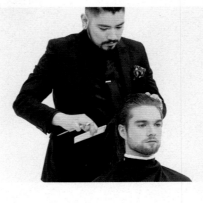

3 Begin by creating a small halo section in the center of the crown. To start the halo, place a diagonal forward parting from the top of each ear across the crown. Then part out a half-circle in front of and behind the diagonal forward parting, forming two semi-circles with the crown at the center. The size of the halo should not extend past the apex and the back of the parietal ridge. Isolate the two semi-circle sections and the hair behind the ear with sectioning clips. Place an additional profile parting from the center of the forehead to the front of the halo parting.

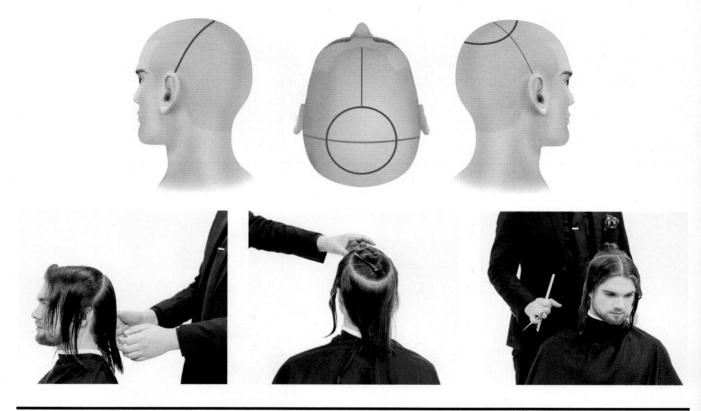

4 Start your traveling guide, by taking a ½-inch (1.3-cm) wide band section from the center of the forehead to the front of the halo section. Elevate the hair straight up from the head at 90 degrees and cut your layers approximately 4 to 5 inches (10.2 to 12.7 cm) in length.

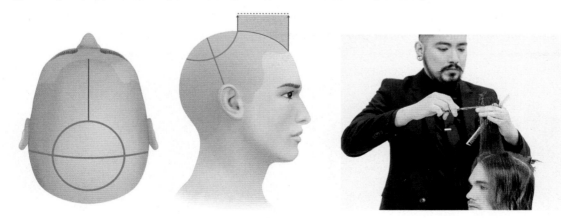

5 On your dominant side, create a ½-inch (1.3-cm) wide, horizontal subsection, from just behind the sideburn to the middle of your guide. Elevate the hair straight up at 90 degrees and cut, following your guide from the previous section.

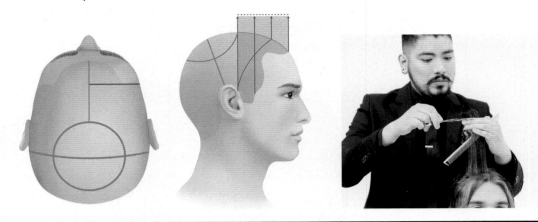

6 Working your way to the back, take another ½-inch (1.3-cm) wide, horizontal subsection, elevate the hair straight up at 90 degrees, and cut, following your guide from the previous section. Continue this technique until you reach the parting at the top of the ear.

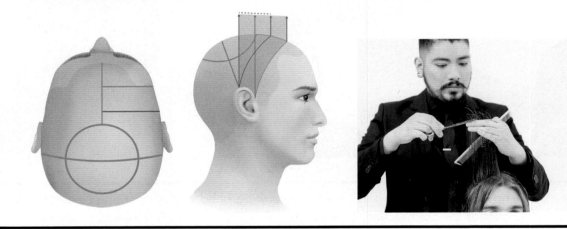

7 When you reach the parting at the top of the ear, switch body positions and repeat on the opposite side, starting just behind the sideburn. After you cut your first subsection, check your balance with the opposite side before continuing. Make any adjustments and continue until you reach the parting at the top of the ear.

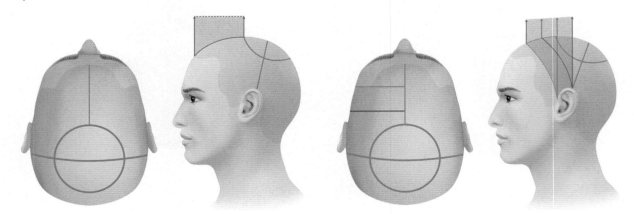

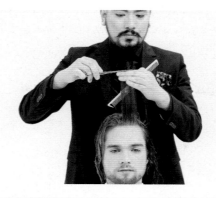

8. Cross-check for balance at the top of the ear, then switch body positions and move back to the side where you started. Here you will release the hair behind the ear and continue cutting, until you reach the center back. To ensure consistency in your cutting line and elevation, subdivide your subsections as you work, following and traveling with your guide from the previously cut section.

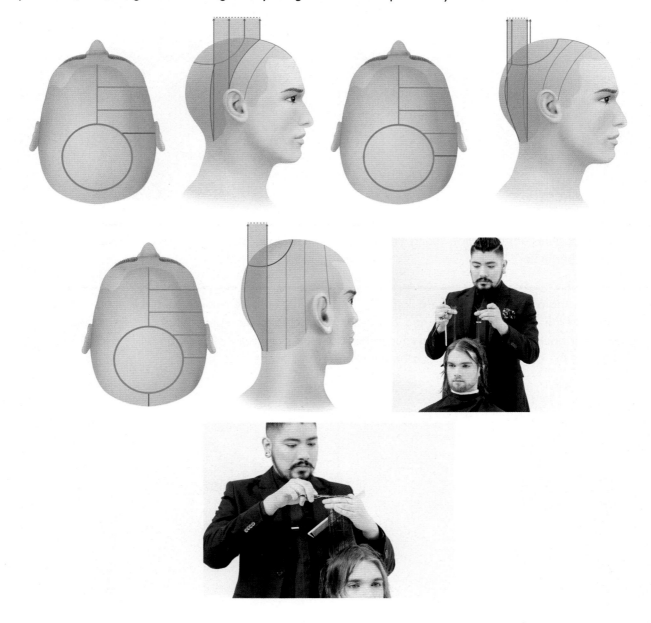

9 When you have reached the center back, switch body positions and repeat the same technique on the opposite side, resuming at the parting at the top of the ear.

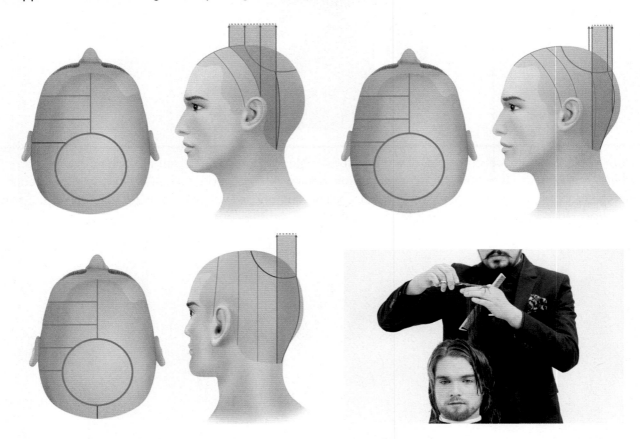

10 Cross-check every third section along with your balance. Your layering will establish your length at the back and perimeter.

11 Release the halo section and take a ½-inch (1.3-cm) wide, profile section from the center of the forehead to the nape. Elevate the hair out at 90 degrees and cut your layers with the round of the head, from back to front, following your guide from the previously cut section underneath. Follow your guide from the previously cut section below and in front of the halo section.

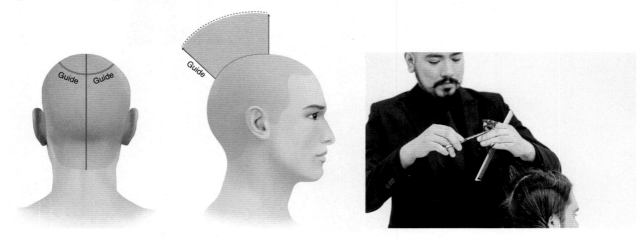

12 When the profile section is complete, create an arc section by taking a curved parting from the top of each ear across the crown and a straight parting from the top of each ear through the occipital.

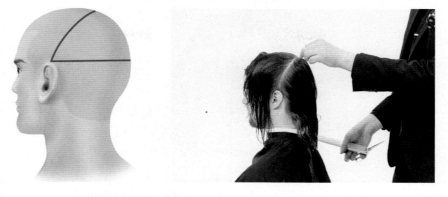

13 At the top of the arc, take a ½-inch (1.3-cm) wide, pivoting section extending to the occipital. Elevate the hair out at 90 degrees and cut your layers with the round of the head, following your guide from the previously cut section.

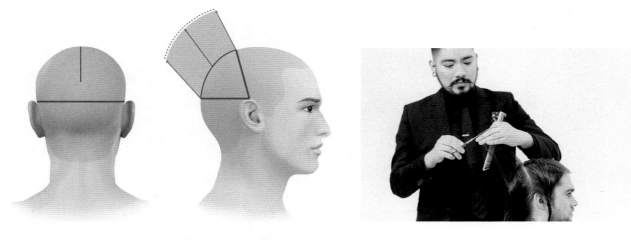

14 Continue taking ½-inch (1.3-cm) wide, pivoting subsections, elevating the hair straight out at 90 degrees, and cutting your layers with the round of the head, following and traveling with your guide from the previous section.

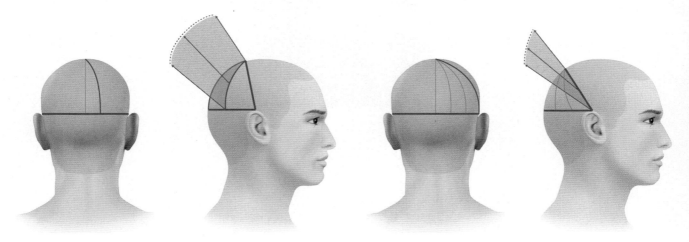

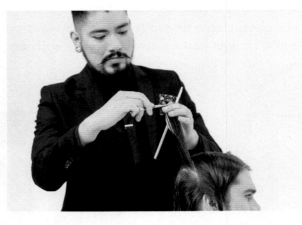

15 Once you reach the parting at the ear, switch body positions and repeat the same technique on the opposite side, starting in the center back and working your way toward the top of the ear.

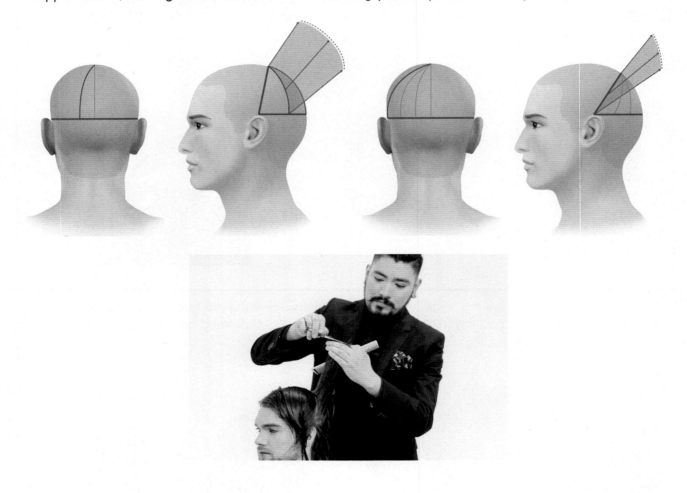

16 Moving in front of the ear, continue taking ½-inch (1.3-cm) wide, pivoting subsections from the crown through to the previously cut section below the guide.

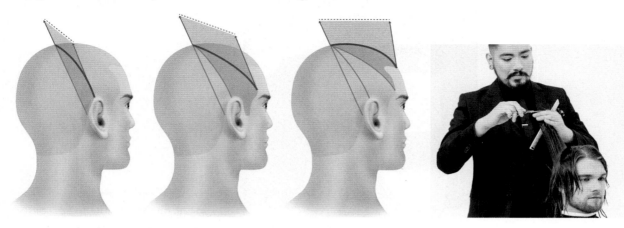

17 Continue this technique until you reach the profile section, then switch body positions and repeat on the opposite side. Begin at the parting at the ear again, and work up to the profile section.

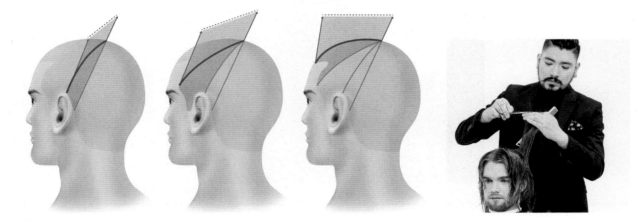

18 Once you complete this technique, cross-check your sections for balance.

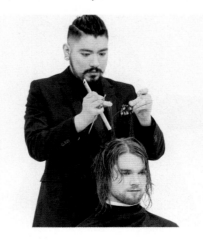

19 When dry, comb all the hair to natural fall and clean up the length and perimeter.

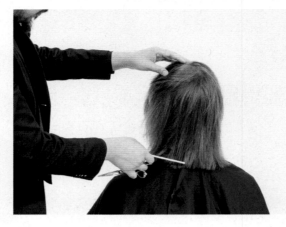

20 Texturize the length and perimeter with point cutting. The line should be textured but not too softened – it is important to keep an element of strength when texturizing men's haircuts.

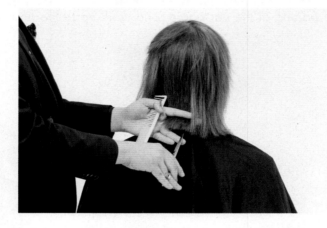

21 In the interior, use notching and free-hand slicing to achieve a shattered effect to the texture. The bang area can be left longer to allow for options, or broken up for a textured look. Perform a fringe consultation and cut the bangs as desired.

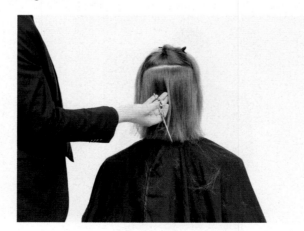

FINISH DESCRIPTION

Your end result will resemble the shag haircut. This shape is ideal for the fashion-forward male; however, the approach can be used on both male and female guests. Texturizing and detailing will give the shape movement and versatility, and ensure that it can be worn casually or styled.

FINISH PREPARATION

When it comes to styling this shape, use a classic styling brush for a styled look or your fingers for a lived-in look. Products of choice for this look are light-hold gel (for control and a wet look), wax (for a matte finish and texture), or texturizing pomade (for an edgier, disheveled look).

STEPS TO FINISH

22 Apply a light-hold gel and thermal protectant, comb through for even distribution.

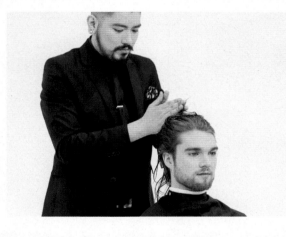

23 Blowdry straight and smooth with a paddle brush or your fingers, depending on how smooth of a finish is desired. Finish by applying a wax to achieve a matte finish and to expose the texture.

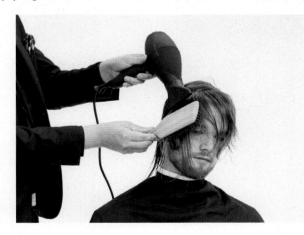

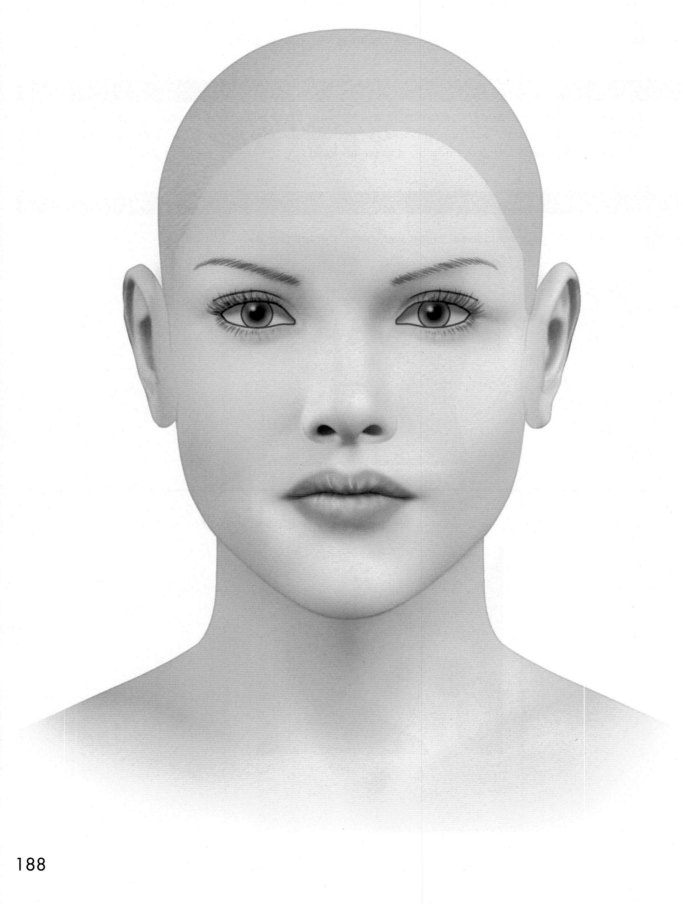

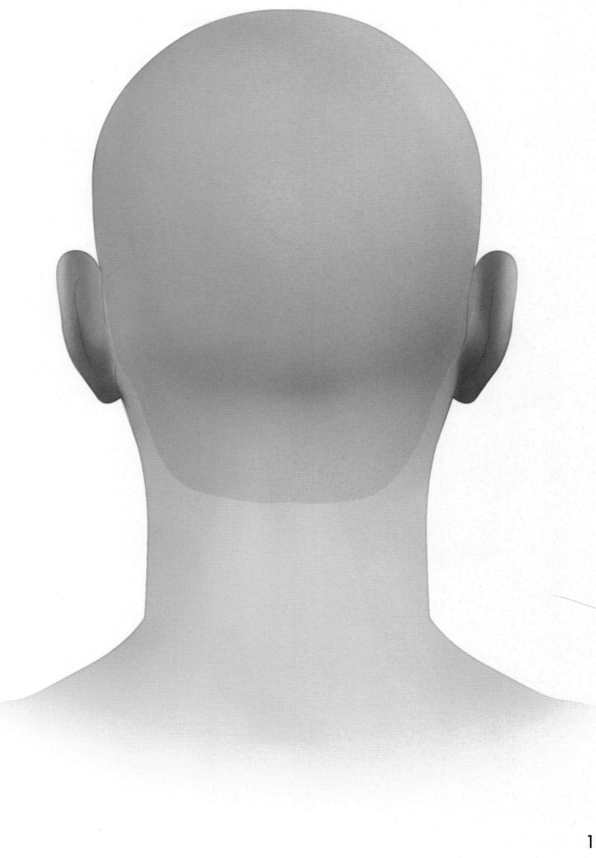

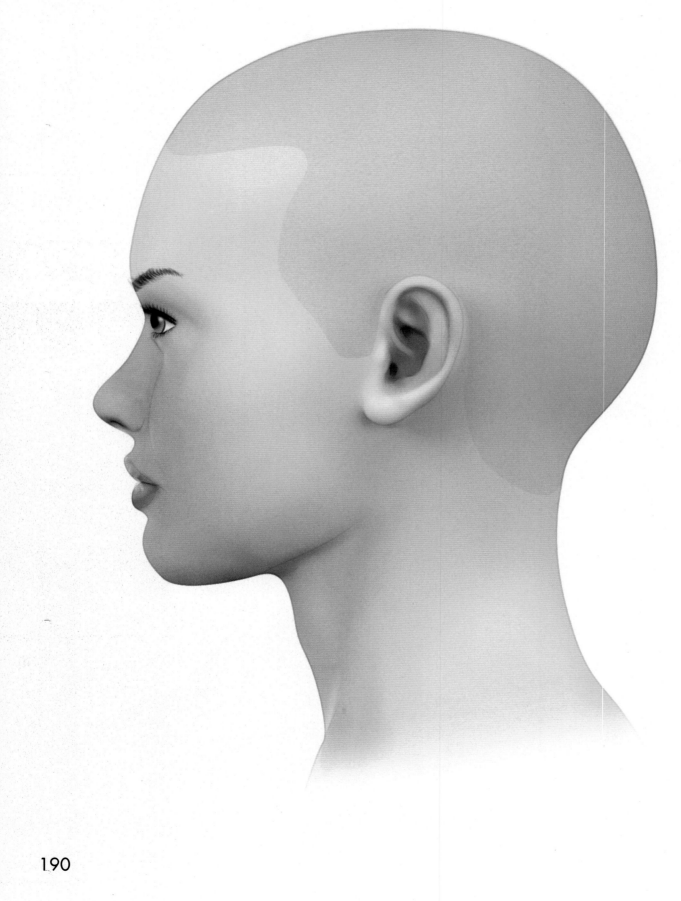

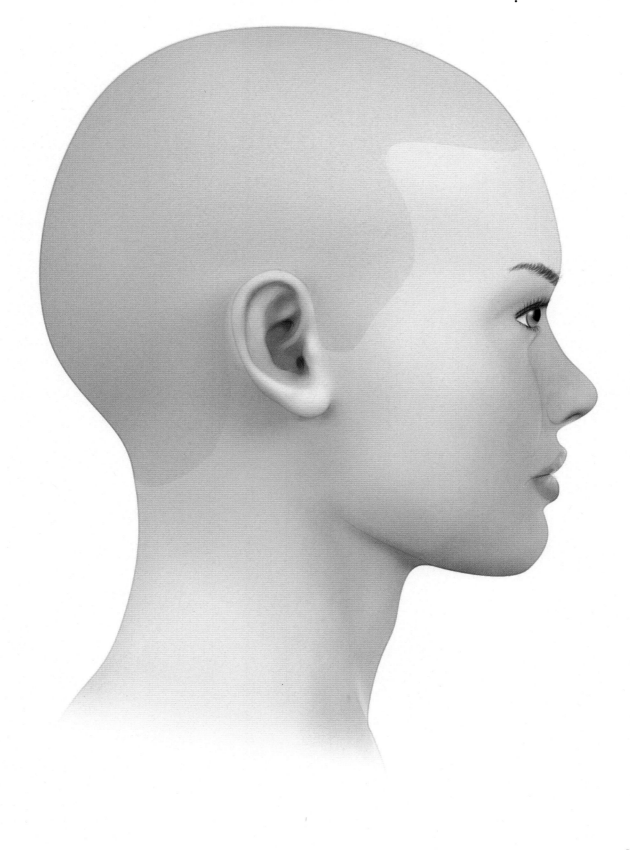

.

HEADSHEETS WOMEN

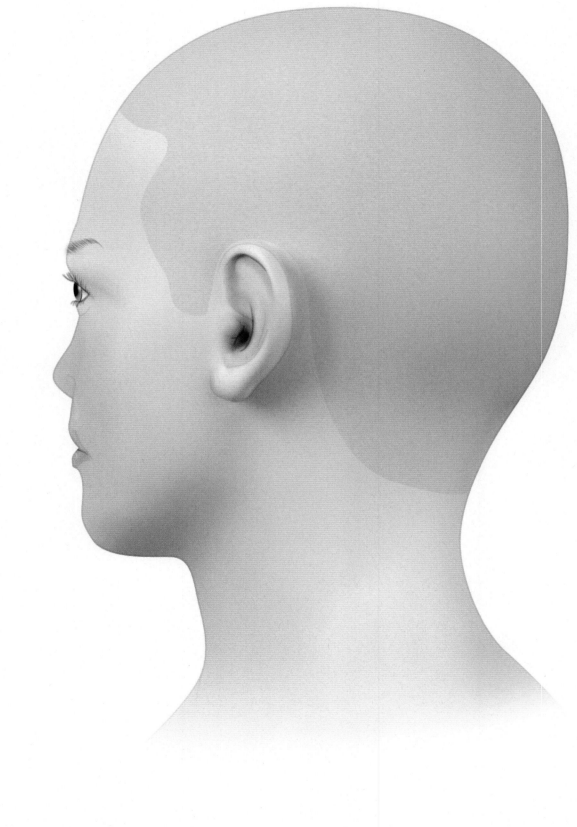

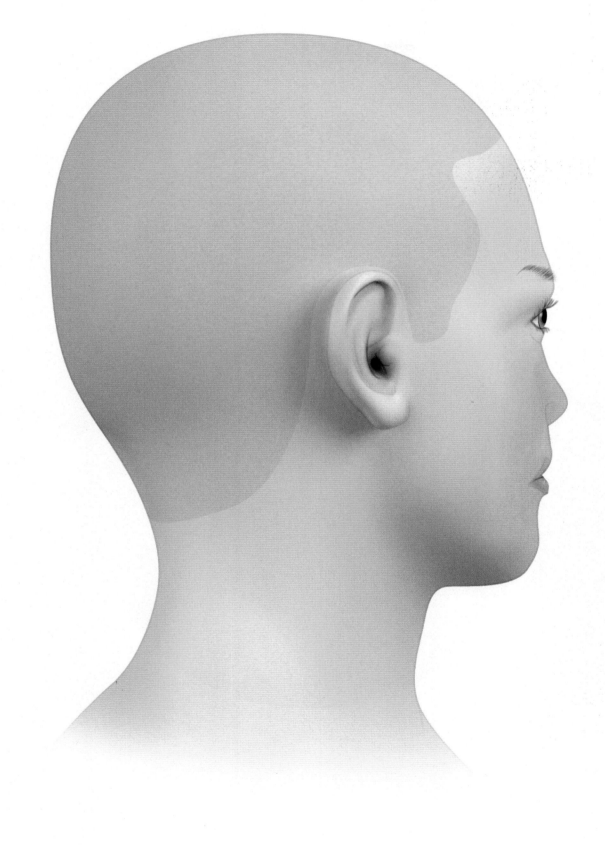

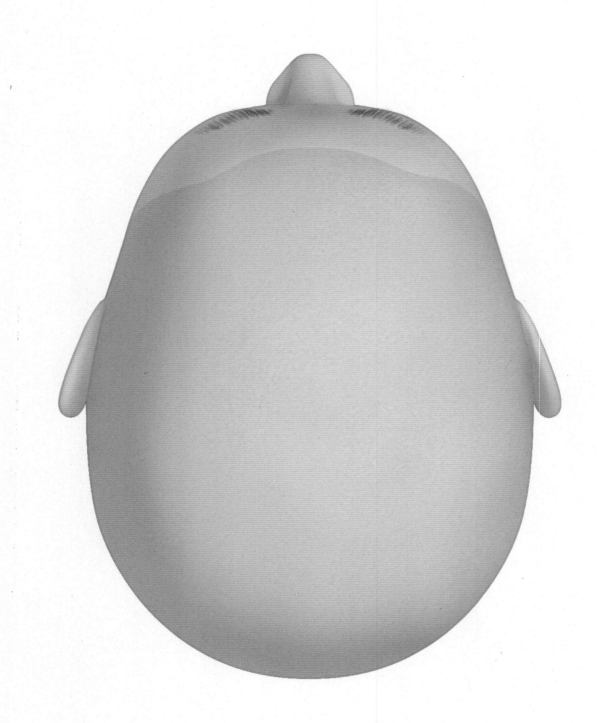

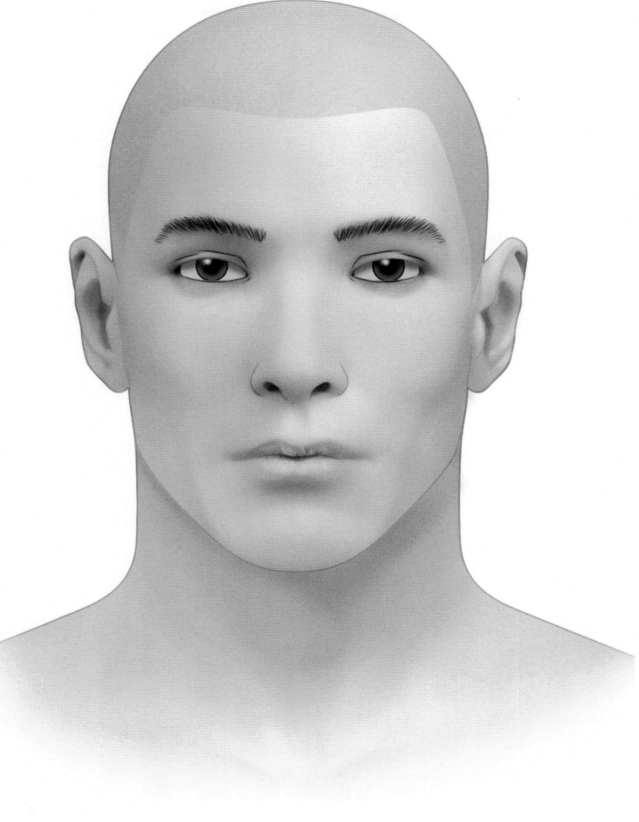

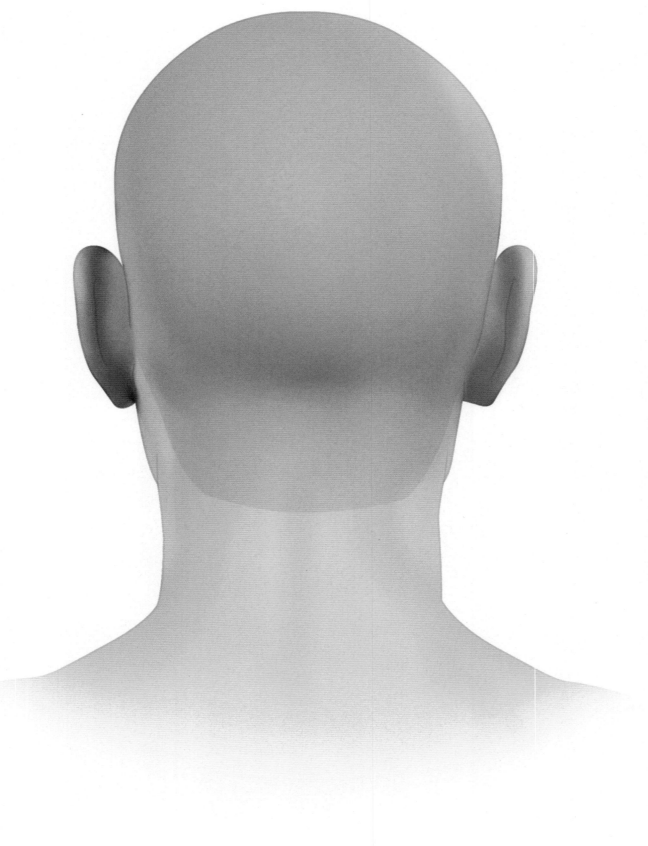

HEADSHEETS MEN

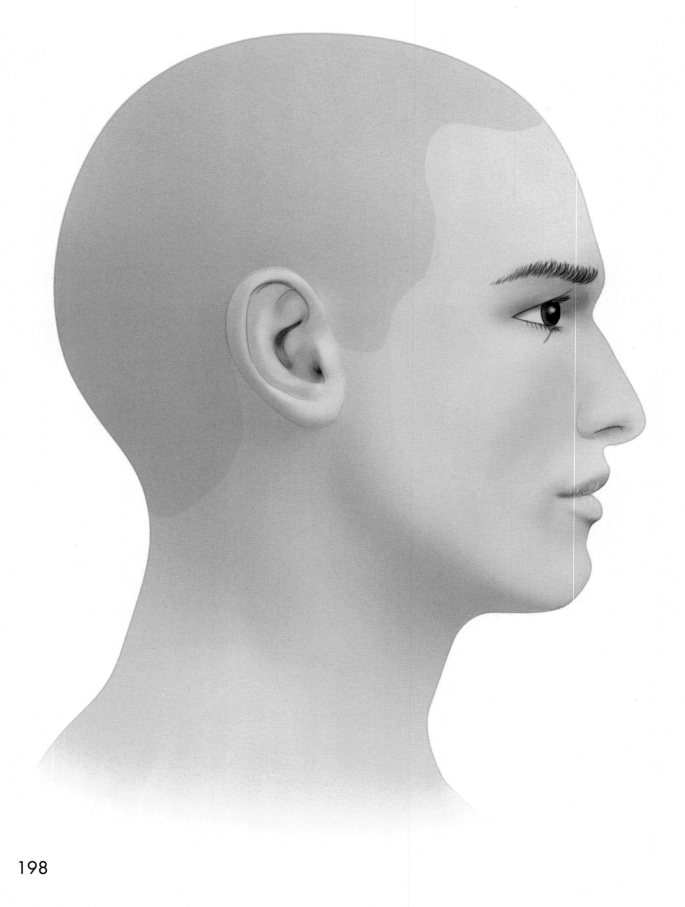

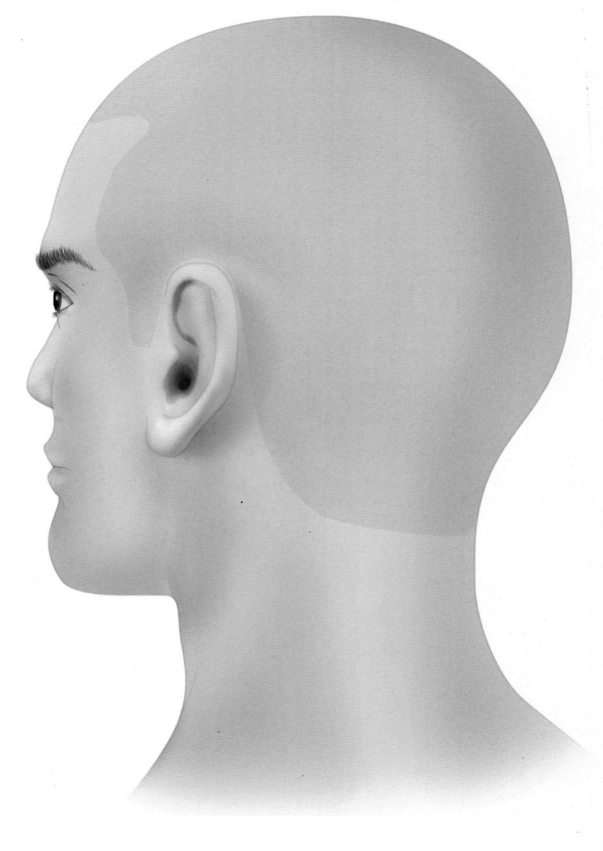

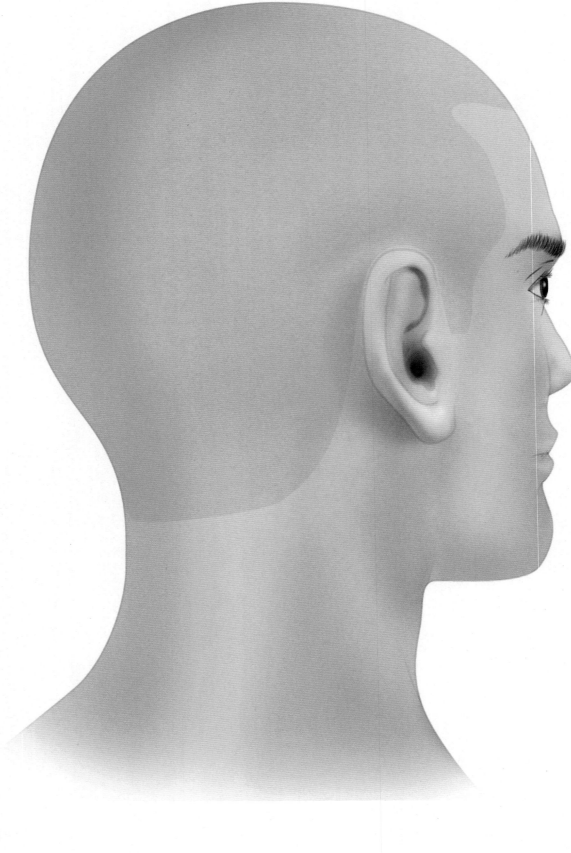

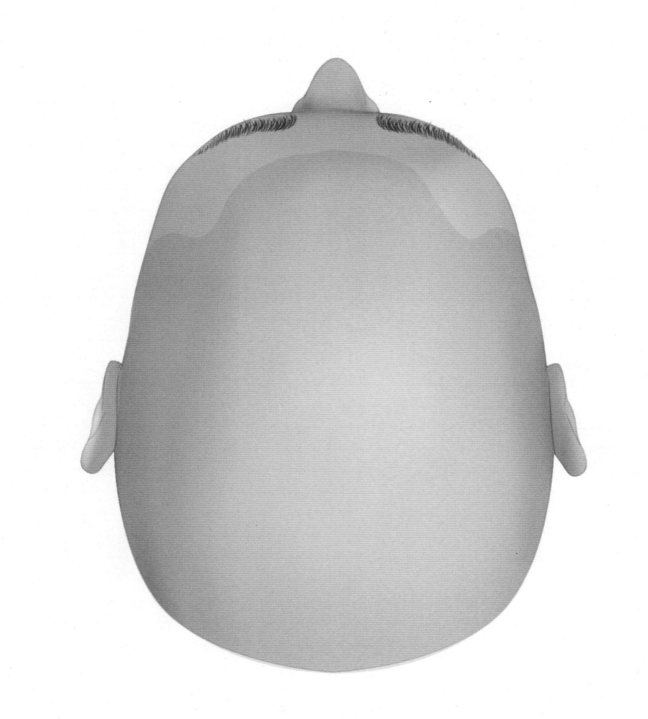

NOTES

NOTES

NOTES